Health and Wellbeing for Babies and Children

This evidence-based text explores children's health and wellbeing from birth to adolescence, taking into account the familial, cultural, social, economic, environmental and global contexts of their lives.

Divided into three parts, this book draws on an international body of research and theoretical perspectives on the determinants of health, such as hereditary, socioeconomic, environmental, geopolitical, gender and cross-cultural factors. It begins with an overview of child health and wellbeing before exploring global influences on health. The second part of the book focuses on health promotion and safeguarding. The final part looks at a range of health conditions that may impact children's health, including infectious diseases, chronic health conditions and mental health. The book ends with a discussion of the role and contribution of families, carers, health professionals, hospitals, the wider community, charities and government, and examines how children with health needs and their families can best be supported. Each chapter includes critical questions, case studies and reflection points, all followed by a commentary to help the reader to think through the issues.

Designed for all those working with children, or studying to work with children, *Health and Wellbeing for Babies and Children: Contemporary Issues* is ideal for students undertaking courses on public health nursing, children's nursing, early years education, childhood studies and social work, among others.

Jackie Musgrave is Associate Head of School, with responsibility for Learning and Teaching, and is part of the Early Childhood team at the Open University, UK.

Health and Wellbeing for Babies and Children

Contemporary Issues

Jackie Musgrave

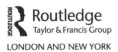
Routledge
Taylor & Francis Group

LONDON AND NEW YORK

Cover image: © Getty Images

First published 2023
by Routledge
4 Park Square, Milton Park, Abingdon, Oxon OX14 4RN

and by Routledge
605 Third Avenue, New York, NY 10158

Routledge is an imprint of the Taylor & Francis Group, an informa business

British Library Cataloguing-in-Publication Data
A catalogue record for this book is available from the British Library

Library of Congress Cataloging-in-Publication Data
Names: Musgrave, Jackie, author.
Title: Health and wellbeing for babies and children: contemporary issues / Jackie Musgrave.
Description: Milton Park, Abingdon, Oxon; New York, NY: Routledge, 2023. | Includes bibliographical references and index.
Identifiers: LCCN 2022020717 (print) | LCCN 2022020718 (ebook) | ISBN 9781032186245 (hardback) | ISBN 9781032186238 (paperback) | ISBN 9781003255437 (ebook)
Subjects: LCSH: Children--Health and hygiene. | Infants--Health and hygiene. | Public health nursing.
Classification: LCC RJ101 .M87 2023 (print) | LCC RJ101 (ebook) | DDC 618.92--dc23/eng/20220625
LC record available at https://lccn.loc.gov/2022020717
LC ebook record available at https://lccn.loc.gov/2022020718

ISBN: 978-1-032-18624-5 (hbk)
ISBN: 978-1-032-18623-8 (pbk)
ISBN: 978-1-003-25543-7 (ebk)

DOI: 10.4324/9781003255437

Typeset in Times New Roman
by MPS Limited, Dehradun

This book is dedicated to all of our precious children in the world, and especially to Ciara, Oscar and Phoebe.

Contents

Figures

Tables

Acknowledgements

My heartfelt thanks to all practitioners and students whose knowledge and contributions have enriched the content of this book.

My thanks to Jude for allowing me to include his baby-led weaning experience.

I acknowledge Carolyn Silberfeld's contribution to the original concept of this book.

Part I

Setting the scene for understanding the complex factors that affect child health

1   Introduction

Introduction

Until about 70 years ago, it was very common for children to die in infancy. During the last century, there have been many medical advances, improvements to the environment, as well as other factors that have improved survival rates of babies and children. Examples of medical advances that have contributed to better survival rates include improved ante-natal and neonatal care for babies before and after birth. The development and availability of surgery and safer anaesthetics mean that there is a wide range of lifesaving and life-improving health care procedures available for babies and small children. Infectious diseases were a cause of death, disability and poor health for babies and young children; however, the discovery of antibiotics has meant that there is treatment available for some bacterial infections that were previously untreatable. Childhood immunisations have contributed to the reduction and in some cases, the elimination of many of the viruses and bacteria that caused communicable diseases that frequently were a cause of death or disability for babies and young children. Also, there have been advances in the medications that can reduce the symptoms of chronic health conditions, for example, inhalers for managing asthma and the availability of injectable insulin for managing diabetes mellitus.

Despite the medical advances that have contributed to improvements in the health of babies and children in many but not all parts of the world, there are many factors that are having a negative impact on their health. For example, there are social, cultural, religious, ethnic characteristics, genetic inheritance, economic, political and geographical influences that interplay and can have a negative or positive impact on children's health. The biggest negative influencing factor on children's health is whether a child lives in poverty, and put simply, the greater the level of poverty experienced, the poorer the child's health. It is important to acknowledge that the aforementioned factors do not occur in isolation, there is intersectionality between these factors. An example from the UK is that children who are from ethnic minority communities are more likely to live in families who have lower incomes, and there may be cultural or religious factors that can be barriers to them accessing health services for their children, all of which can have a negative outcome on children's health.

Despite the medical advances that have contributed to saving lives and improved health for children, since 2016, progress in improving children's health has stalled, and according to a report by the Nuffield Foundation (Oppenheim et al. 2021) in some cases it has reversed. This can be attributable to many reasons. For instance,

DOI: 10.4324/9781003255437-2

the improvements in antenatal and neonatal care have meant that many babies who inherit a genetic condition may survive, whereas only a few years ago, they would not have survived. However, many are born with congenital abnormalities which often leave a legacy of complex medical needs. Consequently, there is an increasing number of children with complex medical needs who require support with their health needs and in turn, with their wellbeing. The global pandemic caused by the coronavirus that started in 2019 has impacted on children's lives and health in a myriad of ways (UNICEF 2021), some examples of the impact will be addressed throughout the book.

The current situation in relation to the health of babies and young children is a complex picture, and this book is intended to help to unravel some of these complexities. Increasing knowledge and understanding of children's health can help to increase confidence about what professionals in children's services can do to play a part in improving the health of children.

Scope of the book

In this book, different aspects of children's health and wellbeing are identified and discussed in detail within the chapters. The chapters give examples of global perspectives on health and wellbeing, acknowledging that access to appropriate health care can be a barrier to improving good health for children. The content of the book is not intended to be exhaustive, or to explain health conditions in detail because there are other sources where such information can be found. However, it is intended to be a provocation to encourage thinking about children's health in the context of their lives. Each baby or child's health needs to be examined from the context of their individual life; it is important to be aware of the factors that can influence their level of health.

Motivation for writing this book

The idea for this book developed from my professional and personal experiences of working with children in different national and international contexts. There was a need to write a book which looked at children's health from a very broad perspective so that it could be relevant for all professionals working with children. Training and working as a nurse and working with children and young people in health and education settings in the UK and in other countries has informed a holistic understanding of how health and wellbeing can impact on children and the adults who care for them. The next section includes some reflections on how my previous experiences can shine a light on the complexities of children's health and wellbeing.

A personal reflection

My professional and personal experiences have informed my position on children's health. Examining my position through the professional lens, I trained as a Registered Children's Nurse and during my paediatric placement as a student, I realised that I wanted to specialise as a children's nurse. Part of my motivation to do this was formed by experiences as a 19-year-old student nurse on a paediatric ward. Many years later, when studying for my master's degree, I carried out research for my dissertation with students to explore their understandings of babies' emotional needs. As I tried to articulate my reflexivity in relation to my choice of research question, I realised that my experiences as a student nurse had left an indelible memory which continued to shape my values and beliefs. This is an excerpt from the research journal I kept when I was conducting my master's research (Musgrave 2009):

> One example to illustrate my sense of unease at practices in hospital at that time that left me bewildered was when I was confidently told by senior staff that babies could not feel pain after surgery and therefore, they did not need analgesia. The appearance of the babies belied the statement. They looked far from comfortable, and I could not understand why this belief was so.

As part of my research for writing this book, I re-visited the textbooks that I referred to in the 1970 and 1980s and I found that none of the content mentions babies' experiences of pain, neither is there discussion of how postoperative pain in babies (or older children) should be managed (Hugh Jolly 1976; June Jolly 1981). A few years later, in 1999, Taylor et al. wrote:

> Infants feel pain, at least many of them scream and try to withdraw from a painful event such as having a blood sample taken. However, circumcision is performed on infant boys quite often without anaesthetic. Marshall (1989) reports that such experiences affect them at the time, both physiologically and psychologically ..., but we do not know what, if any are the long-term effects of painful procedures. (p. 17)

This experience was possibly the foundation of my realisation that there is a need for the professionals who care for babies and children to have a questioning mind about the practices that are seen as acceptable.

I started teaching nursery nurse students in 1996 and quickly became aware of the level of responsibility practitioners are expected to take on in supporting children's health. In 2003, I started to work with Foundation Degree students, who were experienced practitioners. My appreciation deepened about the extent of the role of practitioners working with babies and young children in pre-school education and care settings. They play a key role in supporting children's health, planning around the health needs of children to maximise their participation in routines and activities. What I learned from them shaped my doctoral research. In more recent years, I have become aware of the role that practitioners can and do play in promoting children's health (Musgrave and Payler 2021).

Examining my position on children's health through a personal lens, I have been heavily influenced by my experience as a mother of a child with several interrelated chronic conditions. This experience fed into my reflexivity for choosing to research how practitioners support children with chronic health conditions in early years settings.

In the time that has passed since my experience as a young student nurse back in 1978, our knowledge and views about babies and children have changed, and each profession brings their own perspective to how children's health is viewed. An aim of this book is to encourage you to engage with the information that is included here and to examine the knowledge through your own lens; meaning that you are invited to interpret meaning from your professional and if relevant, your personal perspective. You are encouraged to keep the child and their welfare in mind. However, it is important to be aware that the child is inextricably linked to the context they inhabit. This context may be their educational setting, a health setting and/or social care environment.

A global perspective

The World Health Organisation (WHO) is based in Geneva and was created in 1947, its aim was to bring a unified approach to organising public health. Originally its focus was on reducing the impact of communicable diseases on individuals, but now another important focus is reducing the impact of non-communicable diseases. The WHO is part of the United Nations, which in 1989 produced the Convention on the Rights of the Child, Article 24 of the Rights states:

> the right of the child to the enjoyment of the highest attainable standard of health and to facilities for the treatment of illness and rehabilitation of health. States Parties shall strive to ensure that no child is deprived of his or her right of access to such health care services

The Millennium Development Goals were launched at the start of the new century and were superseded by the Sustainable Development Goals (UNICEF 2018), these are 17 goals to transform our world. Many are designed to improve children's health by addressing the infrastructure of countries, such as access to clean water, but there are specific goals aimed at improving children's health. Many of the goals are inter-related, for example, improving the education of mothers, even to primary level, that is up to the age of 11, has a positive impact on children's health. Partly because increased literacy can mean they are able to access written material relating to health.

The WHO aims to promote the concept of 'Universal Healthcare for All' meaning that people should be able to access the 'promotive, preventive, curative, rehabilitative and palliative health services they need' (WHO 2019) without causing financial hardship.

We live in a global world, and England's Chief Medical Officer's report in 2019, (Davies 2019) stated that she believes that 'the health of people in the UK is increasingly connected with the health of those in other countries' (p. 1). This point is especially pertinent at a time where global events such as the impact of the coronavirus pandemic and migration is at unprecedented levels which illustrate that we need to learn more about the factors that can influence children's health, many of which will be explored in this book. We also need to learn from global initiatives that can help us to improve children's health. Increasing individuals' and organisations' understanding of how health can be promoted is a global aim. My experiences of working in India and in the Gambia gave me valuable experience on my insight into children's health and I have summarised some of my thoughts in the following reflection.

Personal reflection

Educational visits to India and Gambia gave me invaluable insights into the health needs of children in countries without national health services; children are especially vulnerable to the impact of under-developed or a lack of health services. The knowledge I acquired from having the privilege of meeting people who taught me so much, helped me to develop an awareness of children's health from a global perspective. Such an understanding is especially important at a time when the global movement of people between countries around the world is so great because of the impact of war, conflict and economic influences. In addition, families bring with them the social and cultural influences that have shaped their health beliefs, which in turn can sometimes have negative impacts on their children's health. Such beliefs can sometimes clash with ours and may cause ethical tensions and dilemmas. In some circumstances, health beliefs and practices may be illegal, for example, female genital mutilation.

The health of children is highly influenced by the country they live in and in particular the level of income is a significant factor. The World Bank (2019 a and 2019 b) categorises countries as being high, upper-middle, lower-middle and low-income countries. These classifications are used in this book.

Defining health and wellbeing

The World Health Organisation 2022 states that 'health is a state of complete physical, mental and social well-being and not merely the absence of disease or infirmity'. (WHO 2022) This definition suggests that health is affected by many factors that are inter-related and implies that mental health can affect physical health, and vice versa, and the social aspects and the context of where people live. Thus, we can draw from this definition that health is a complex concept. In relation to children, the complexity is even more profound. Kate Leddington, a student I worked with, wrote in an assignment what health in relation to children means to her

> to ensure we provide high levels of structured care viewing the child holistically, understating that their needs are unique meaning individual barriers will need to be removed in order to participate in education. This should be achieved by working directly with the child themselves, their parents and multitude of other services

Kate's definition highlights that children's health is influenced by their environment and the adults who care for them, therefore it is important that health is viewed as a holistic concept which can only be fully understood by exploring and examining the different contexts of children's lives.

Children's health: age and stage of development

This book examines health from different age bands, throughout the book, the terms early childhood to describe babies and young children aged 0–7 years, middle childhood for children aged 8–12 and adolescence for children aged 12–18. However, these age bands are not prescriptive, but are used to illustrate that a child's age and stage of development can be an important influence on their health. Whatever age a child is, they may or may not be able to articulate the impact of experiencing poor, or good, health on their wellbeing. In addition, their age and stage of development can influence how much they understand about health, and it is important that they are involved in decisions. In England, the Ten Year National Service Framework (DH 2004) stated that by 2013 health professionals must involve children and young people in healthcare decisions. According to McPherson (2010) involving children in their care can lead to better outcomes in childhood and in later life. Adolescents' health is of particular concern because every year globally 1.2 million adolescents die, often from preventable causes (The Lancet 2017), however, this age group is often rendered invisible in policies and investment frameworks. In contemporary times, children are involved in healthcare decisions in many spaces. For example, Chitsaben (2018) blogged about the importance of engaging children and young people in the commissioning and delivery of mental health services. However, in many places around the UK and the world, this remains an aspiration.

Contemporary child health issues

Children's health and wellbeing has never been as complex, and it is becoming increasingly controversial. Before exploring why this is so, it may be helpful to summarise the contemporary issues that affect children, these are summarised in Figure 1.1.

The chapters in the book will address the health issues that are currently affecting children in relation to their education, within their home and family as well as examining where they live in the world.

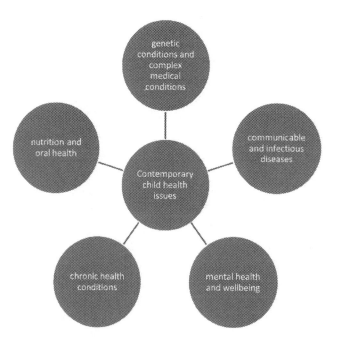

Figure 1.1 Summary of contemporary child health issues.

Structure of the book

This book is divided into three parts. Throughout each part reference is made to children across the age range, using relevant literature and research. These ages are not consistently separated more distinctly because health issues and many of the complexities relating to health tend to be generic, rather than related to specific age groups. Threaded through each chapter are scenarios that relate to the theme of the chapter, accompanying the scenarios are questions which are followed by commentary aimed at provoking thinking and developing the readers' knowledge and understanding.

Parts in the book

The book is divided into three parts:

Part I: Setting the scene for understanding the complex factors that affect child health

In Chapter 1, the aims of the book are outlined, the content of each chapter is summarised and the structure of the book is described.

Chapter 2 sets the scene by discussing the influences on children's health from the perspective of the child; the family or carers; the community where the child lives; as well as the country and global influences.

Chapter 3 looks at the influence and impact of child health screening and surveillance during the pre-conception, ante-natal and early childhood period. An increase in the intake of alcohol during pregnancy is causing a growth in the number of babies who are being born with Foetal Alcohol Syndrome (FAS). However, it is an under-recognised condition that has long-term impact on children; therefore, a case study that focuses on the implications of FAS is included.

Part II: Preventative steps that can be taken to improve the health and wellbeing of children

Chapter 4 focuses on health promotion in relation to children, explaining why it is important to invest in preventing conditions from developing. It defines what is meant by health promotion, and explores the health promotion priorities both nationally and globally. The content summarises the role of professionals in promoting health in children.

Chapter 5 examines how children can be protected from harm and examines safeguarding through a health lens. The content focuses on keeping children safe and highlights the importance of knowing children and their families in order to identify threats to their safety. Some of the ways that the environment can impact on health and wellbeing, such as family circumstances and potential hazards, are explored. Prevention of harm is discussed and safeguarding in the English context is summarised. The vulnerability of children who are looked-after; runaway children; children with Special Educational Needs are touched on. Some of the global safeguarding issues are highlighted and the possible effect on their health and safety are included. Challenges to health as children move into adolescence and risk taking as a common feature of behaviour is explored.

Part III: Supporting children with health conditions *focuses on contemporary conditions that affect children's physical and mental health.*

Chapter 6 examines some of the infectious/communicable diseases that can impact on children's health. It begins by looking at the causes of infections and infestations and then outlines the common preventable infections that commonly affect children. The chapter includes information about tropical communicable and infectious conditions.

The consequences of infectious diseases are also included. Parasitic conditions and the adverse impact they can have on children's health are explored in this chapter.

Chapter 7 looks at the children's mental health and wellbeing. The content includes a discussion about what we mean by 'mental health' and gives an overview of what contributes to the foundation of good mental health in children. For instance, the need for children to develop a sense of belonging in order to have good wellbeing and the importance of managing transitions is discussed. Some of the factors that predispose children to developing mental health conditions are included, such as adverse life experiences, as well as highlighting, grief, loss and bereavement.

Chapter 8 focuses on children's chronic health conditions which include asthma and other respiratory conditions; metabolic conditions such as diabetes mellitus, epilepsy and other neurological conditions; cardiothoracic and circulatory problems; skeletal and orthopaedic conditions: juvenile arthritis; skin conditions, such as eczema are explored. The impact of chronic health conditions on families is highlighted as well as the management of chronic conditions. Some aspects of care relating to the transitions from children to adult health services is covered. The chapter includes a framework for managing the care and education of children with one or more chronic condition.

Chapter 9 is an overview of nutrition and oral health. This chapter develops the content relating to the role of good nutrition and dental care in the prevention of poor overall, going into greater detail of the content in Chapter 4.

Chapter 10 looks at who cares for children's health and wellbeing, exploring the role and contribution of families, carers, education settings, health professionals, hospitals, the wider community, charities and government. it examines the ways in which children's complex health needs and their families can be supported. Within this chapter, some of the complex cases that can occur when parental wishes and medical opinion differ are explored.

Chapter 11 is the final chapter and is a brief summary of the content of the book, encouraging the reader to regard health as integral to children's health and wellbeing, and for them to recognise that everybody has a responsibility to support and promote children's health, encouraging the reader to reflect on how the knowledge they gained from reading the book will help them to improve their practice when working with children and signposting the reader to resources that will help them to continue to keep abreast of knowledge about the complexities of children's health.

Conclusion

I hope you will enjoy this book and that it will help you to develop further your knowledge and understanding of the complexities in children's health and wellbeing and how the contexts of children's lives and experiences can be so pivotal to their future health and wellbeing.

References

Chitsabesan, P. (2018) The importance of engaging children and young people in the commissioning and delivery of mental health services. Blog available from https://www.england.nhs.uk/blog/the-importance-of-engaging-children-and-young-people-in-the-commissioning-and-delivery-of-mental-health-services/, accessed 18 March 2022.

Davies, S. C. (2019) Annual report of the chief medical officer. Health – our global asset. Available from file:///C:/Users/jm39645/Work%20Folders/Documents/Child%20Health/Chief_Medical_Officer_annual_report_2019_-_partnering_for_progress_-_accessible.pdf, accessed 18 March 2022.

Department of Health (2004) Core Standards: National Services Framework for Children, Young People and Maternity Services. London: The Stationery Office.

Jolly, H. (1976) Diseases of Children (3rd Ed). Oxford: Blackwell Scientific Publications.

Jolly, J. (1981) The Other Side of Paediatrics. London: McMillan Press Ltd.

Marshall, R. E. (1989) Neonatal pain associated with caregiving procedures. *Pediatric clinics of North America*, 36(4): 885–903.

McPherson, A. (2010) Involving children: why it matters. In Redsell, S. and Hastings, S. (Eds) Listening to Children and Young People in Healthcare Consultations. Oxford: Radcliffe Publishing.

Musgrave, J. (2009) Don't pick the baby up – she"ll become spoil. Unpublished Masters dissertation. University of Sheffield.

Musgrave, J., and Payler, J. (2021) Proposing a model for promoting Children's Health in Early Childhood Education and Care Settings. Children and Society.

Oppenheim, C., Batchelor, R., Hargreaves, D., Rehill, J., and Shah, R. (2021) Are young children healthier than they were two decades ago? Report in the Changing Faces of Early Childhood in Britain series. Nuffield Foundation. Available from www.Nuffieldfoundation. org, published 9 December 2021.

Taylor, J., Muller, D., Wattley, L., and Harris, P. (1999) Nursing Children: Psychology, Research and Practice (3rd Ed). Cheltenham: Stanley Thornes.

The Lancet (2017) Comment: where is the accountability to adolescents? Available from https://www.thelancet.com/journals/lancet/article/PIIS0140-6736(17)32482-0/fulltext, accessed 26 July 2019.

The World Health Organisation (2022) Health and Wellbeing Available from https://www.who.int/data/gho/data/major-themes/health-and-well-being. accessed 17 July 2022.

The World Bank (2019a) Classifying countries by income. Available from http://datatopics.worldbank.org/world-development-indicators/stories/the-classification-of-countries-by-income.html, accessed 26 July 2019.

The World Bank (2019b) Classifying countries by income. Available from https://datatopics.worldbank.org/world-development-indicators/stories/the-classification-of-countries-by-income.html, accessed 7 September 2019.

UNICEF (2021) Covid 19 and children. Available from https://data.unicef.org/covid-19-and-children/, accessed 18 March 2022.

UNICEF (2018) Unicef and the sustainable development goals.

United Nations Human Rights (1989) Convention on the rights of the child. Available from http://www.ohchr.org/EN/ProfessionalInterest/Pages/CRC.aspx, accessed 6 April 2018.

2 Influences affecting and impacting on the health and wellbeing of children

Introduction

This chapter explores the factors that can affect all children's mental and physical health. To understand the contemporary state of children's health, it is important to explore some of the influences on children's health from a historical perspective to gain an understanding of how the factors have or in some cases have not changed. The influences on children's health in contemporary times are complex and, in an attempt, to simplify the factors, Figure 2.1 illustrates the factors as 'layers' within the child's environment. Each of the layers examines the following perspectives:

1   The child
2   The family or carers
3   The child's community including education settings
4   The country a child lives in
5   The global factors that impact on children's health.

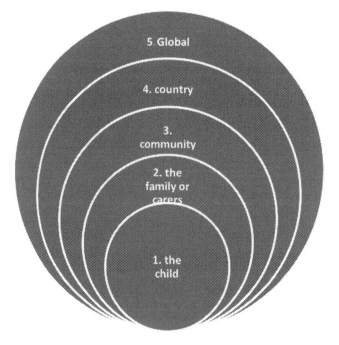

Figure 2.1 The layers in a child's environment that affect mental and physical health.

DOI: 10.4324/9781003255437-3

However, it is important to bear in mind that the layers cannot be distinct because the factors overlap and interrelate, these points will be explained in greater detail later in the chapter.

Historical context

In the 1850s, the time around childbirth and the first year of life was especially dangerous for children's health. In addition, living conditions were squalid for most poor people, the presence of sewerage in the street and an absence of clean water meant that infectious diseases were a significant cause of death and disability. The mortality rate for children before the age of 5 was high, many succumbed to life-threatening health problems. As many as 50% of babies in cities died before their first birthday (Horn 1974). In England in the 1850s, the opening of hospitals dedicated to meeting the health care needs of children was a significant landmark in recognising that children had different health needs and were not simply small adults. The hospitals were built in poverty-stricken areas of London, Birmingham and other industrial cities, reflecting the fact that children who live in poverty are more likely to experience poor health than better-off children.

At the start of the last century, in the 1900s, one in six infants did not live until their first birthday, meaning that the infant mortality rate was around 150–160 per 1,000 live births. In 1919, the McMillan sisters opened their nursery schools in England, this was the start of a trend of using education settings as a place where children's health could be improved, a trend which continues today. The 20th century was a time where there were significant advances that contributed to increased numbers of children surviving the first year of life, as well as improving their health.

The contemporary context globally

Despite the improvements in medical care and living conditions which have made positive improvements to children's health, there are global concerns about the state of children's health. The Royal College of Paediatrics and Child Health (RCPCH) in their 2017 report, the State of Child Health in the four nations of the UK, points out that during the last century there has been considerable investment to promote children's health. Currently, infant mortality is 3.9 per 1,000, meaning that 1 in 256 infants do not reach their first birthday. Despite these improvements, the UK mortality rate for children is higher than in other comparable countries. In contrast, child mortality in Sub-Saharan Africa in 2013 was estimated to be 92 deaths per 1,000 live births. It is important to bear in mind that in all countries of the world, whatever the level of income, there are significant numbers of people who live in poverty. Living in poverty is a significant determinant of health worldwide and 'children are more affected by socio-economic circumstances than any other age group in society' (Blair et al. 2010, p. 77). Food insecurity is a factor that impacts on many children regardless of where they live. Some of the causes of poor child health have changed with the passage of time, it remains the case that poor nutrition, diarrhoeal diseases, and some infections remain significant threats to their health and are more common in children who are poor (Blair et al. 2010). The global pandemic that started in 2019 has had significant impacts on the physical and mental health of many babies and young children. The Sustainable Development Goal Report (UN 2020) estimates that the economic impact of the pandemic will push 71 million people back into extreme poverty.

The contemporary context in high-income countries

In high and some mid-income countries, improvements in sanitation and health services have had the effect of reducing the number of children who die from communicable diseases. For more than 100 years, there have been sustained improvements in the mortality rate of newborn babies. Unfortunately, despite the efforts of many high-income countries to improve the health of children the infant mortality decline has plateaued (Royal College of Paediatrics and Child Health 2018). The contemporary issues that affect babies' and children's health are summarised in Table 2.1.

The contemporary context in mid- and low-income countries

The contemporary issues that impact disproportionately on low- and middle-income countries are infectious diseases and maternal and child health. The period of life around birth, the neonatal period (0–28 days) is still a vulnerable period and children

Table 2.1 A summary of contemporary child health issues

Child health issue	Examples of conditions and/ or causes of conditions	Comment
Genetic conditions and complex medical conditions	Poor ante-natal health care, inherited conditions; birth trauma	Many babies survive pregnancy and childbirth but may have complex medical needs and/or disabilities (see Chapter 3 for more detail)
Communicable and infectious diseases	Viruses and bacteria parasites	Many communicable diseases are avoidable by immunisation and infection control measures (see Chapter 6 for more detail)
Mental health and wellbeing	Anxiety, depression, post-traumatic stress disorder	It is estimated that there has been a 5-fold increase in mental health problems since 1998 (see Chapter 7 for more detail)
Chronic health conditions	Asthma, diabetes mellitus, sickle cell disease	Chronic health conditions can be managed with correct treatment, but can still be a cause of child mortality (see Chapter 8 for more detail)
Nutrition and dental health	Obesity Inadequate nutrition Poor oral health	Increased levels of obesity are a global problem. Deprived boys most likely to be obese (see Chapter 9)

living in poverty in low-income countries are more likely to die than newborns in higher-income countries. As many as 44% of all child deaths occur in this period; many of these deaths are because of difficulties at birth and with the relevant support, it is estimated that two of three deaths are preventable (Williams et al. 2016).

The cause of poor child health and deaths in low-income countries is still mostly because of infectious diseases, with diarrhoea and pneumonia being the leading causes of death in babies and older children. There has been significant progress in reducing the ways that malaria affects children's health, largely because of the use of insecticide-treated bed nets by children living in sub-Saharan Africa where malaria is endemic.

Nutrition is a cause of poor child health and obesity in childhood is a problem in low-income countries as well as inadequate food availability causing children to be underweight and malnourished. Malnutrition can leave children susceptible to infections.

The evidence for supporting and promoting child health

Supporting and promoting good health for children from conception and in the early years is of benefit not just during childhood, but across the lifespan. Additionally, Heckman, the economics professor's widely reported evidence describes how investment in the early years, including services for children's health has economic benefits across society (Heckman 2022). Marmot (2015) examined the links between poverty and health, and he outlined the importance of investment in supporting children's development in the early years:

> child development matters hugely for subsequent health and health equity, and that good early child development is shaped by the environment in which children grow and develop. (p. 142)

Marmot's assertion about the importance of the child's environment in relation to their health serves as a reminder to all of us that we have a responsibility to make a positive contribution to the factors in their environment that influence children's physical and mental health.

Examining the factors that influence children's physical and mental health

Figure 2.1 illustrates the many factors that influence children's health. At the heart of the diagram is the child and each layer represents other influences that are within the child's family, community, country and the planet.

Factors within the child

Pre-conception, pregnancy and childbirth

There are numerous factors that can influence the child's health even before conception and during pregnancy. These factors include lifestyle choices such as the quality of their diet, whether the mother smokes, drinks alcohol or takes illegal drugs; these factors are discussed in more detail in Chapter 3. Childbirth is safer than it was in the past, this is partly because ante-natal care is provided to pregnant women in many countries; however, such care is not available to or accessed by all mothers. Giving birth remains a time when babies are vulnerable to trauma, for example, lack of oxygen to the brain can cause damage that can result in cerebral palsy.

Genetics

Each cell of the human body contains the genes that a child inherits from their parents is a powerful influence on their health. The genetic material that a baby receives from their biological parents can predispose them to inherit a condition that affects their health in a myriad of ways. There are many inherited conditions and depending on what the condition is, this can mean that a child may have complex or additional needs right from birth. An inherited condition such as Noonan or Down Syndrome can be apparent in the very early days of life. Cystic fibrosis is another inherited condition; however, the signs may not emerge until the baby is a few months old. There are conditions that can develop later in childhood, such as asthma or diabetes, these conditions are discussed in Chapter 8. And there are conditions that are passed on that may not emerge until adulthood, such as heart disease. Also genetic conditions that cause health conditions, a baby's individual temperament can influence the development of their approach to life, this in turn can impact on wellbeing and in the longer term, this can impact on mental health.

Disability and complex medical needs

Babies and children may develop a disability or a long-term legacy because of genetic inheritance, because of their experience before or during birth or as a result of an infection or injury. For some children, the effects or disability can be so extensive that they have complex medical needs. Having complex needs or a disability can be a factor that predisposes children to poor health, such as being vulnerable to infections.

Age

A child's age has a profound impact on the state of their health. Babies and children under the age of 2 are especially vulnerable to the causes of poor or less than optimal health. This is partly because of their immature immune systems, their ability to articulate their feelings and symptoms to adults, and critically because adults may fail to recognise when a baby is unwell and needs attention. The impact on babies' health because of the pandemic restrictions which led to a reduction, or no, health services being available to them. The lack of regard of babies and young children's welfare during this period has been described as a 'baby blind spot' (Parent Infant Partnership 2021) meaning that they were over-looked. The consequences of lack of attention to the health of our youngest citizens because of the restrictions imposed are likely to have impact in childhood and possibly across the age span. Certainly, there has been an increase in cases of child abuse which was especially prevalent in the youngest age group, this is highlighted in Chapter 4.

As children move into adolescence, they may have more autonomy about some of their life choices and this can be positive or negative. However, for some adolescents, this can be a life stage which brings additional risks, globally there are many who are homeless, and they live on the streets, thus they face additional health challenges and risks to their safety as discussed in Chapter 5. Adolescent health is an area that requires more attention.

A child's view of health: Oscar, aged 8

Children shape their own view of what health means to them, and it can be revealing to ask children what their views are about health because they can have very well thought through ideas. Oscar, aged 8, was asked the following questions (Figure 2.2):

1   What does health mean to you, Oscar?
    Oscar: Health to me means that it is a source of life, so people live without things like cancer.
2   How do you stay healthy?
    Oscar: Doing 1 hour's exercise and eating plenty of meat, protein, veg and oranges. Having exercise and healthy food.
3   What makes you feel unhealthy?
    Oscar: Too much sweets and chocolate.
4   How do you feel when you are unwell?
    Oscar: It makes me feel very droopy and hot.
5   What does the school do to improve your health?
    Oscar: Improves my knowledge and wellbeing.

Asking Oscar these questions gives some insight into some of the factors that have influenced his view of health. Oscar has made a clear connection between being healthy and the absence of diseases, such as cancer. Perhaps he has experience of a family member who had cancer, or perhaps he has become aware of the condition on television adverts. He also makes connections between the importance of promoting his health by taking exercise. He has been specific about the importance of healthy eating and was able to differentiate between food that he regards as being healthy and unhealthy, specifying the need to avoid 'too much sweets and chocolate'. Oscar associated feeling unwell with his experience of having what was probably an infection which made him 'feel very droopy and hot'. His response to being asked about what he thought his school does to improve his health was of particular note. This is because he was asked these questions at the start of the summer break which had just started after 15 months of disruption and school closures. It is especially noteworthy that Oscar made a connection with being at school and his knowledge and wellbeing.

From this brief exchange, we can surmise that Oscar has formed his view of health by making connections with what he has learned from factors within the context of his life. He has more than likely been influenced by the adults around him, and the media.

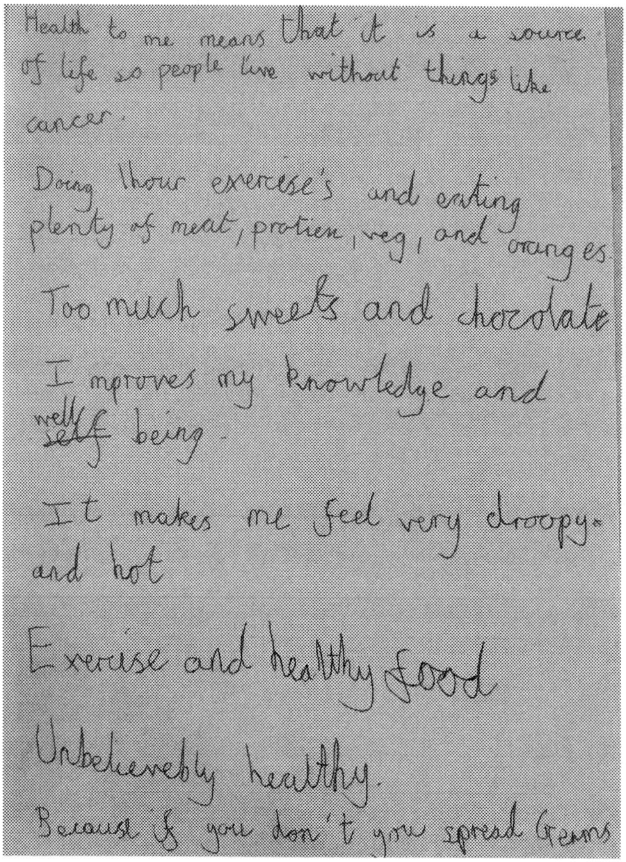

Figure 2.2 Oscar's thoughts about what health means to him.

And importantly, he appears to have been influenced by his school environment and recognised that being at school improved his knowledge and wellbeing. You may draw other conclusions from Oscar's responses.

Activity

Perhaps you would like to do a similar exercise and ask children these questions. Consider asking children of similar or different ages.

What are the differences or similarities between their responses?

How do their insights help to increase your awareness about children's views of health?

Factors within the family

The family that a child is born into has a profound influence on children's health. As humans, we all have basic needs that must be met, these include nutrition, sleep, rest, exercise and so on, such basic needs are the foundation for good physical and mental health. Babies and young children need adults who can provide the daily routines that include opportunities for them to receive the physical basic needs. Demonstrating love and affection helps to promote attachment and the development of positive relationships that are the foundation of good wellbeing and positive mental health. For many children, the family is where they will receive the daily routine care that is the foundation of good physical and mental health. However, some families are unable to provide a routine that meets their children's, and some families live in 'household chaos' which is defined by Khatiwada et al. (2018) as 'chaotic living due to high levels of disorganization, over crowdedness, noise, lack of routine and unpredictability in daily activities' (p. 6). Khatiwada et al go on to state that families living in chaos can make a significant contribution to children's poor health. In particular, their study found that there was an association between chaos and increased weight gain in babies at the age of 12 months.

The level of education of the parents, especially the mother's level of education is a significant factor on children's health (Marmot 2010). This fact is illustrated in a World Health Organisation report which stated that babies with mothers who had secondary education were more likely to survive than babies with mothers who had no education (Marmot 2015). This can be attributed to the ways that literacy and access to digital resources that parents can seek information about children's health.

Parenting style

The way that children are parented can have a direct impact on children's health. Baumrind (1966) described parents as being authoritative (nurturing, responsive and supportive); authoritarian (expect orders to be obeyed without question); permissive (a lack of boundaries) or neglectful (not meeting children's needs). As always, applying one model to all children and families is not helpful because there is a multitude of factors that can influence how parents approach the rearing of their children. For example, what is culturally acceptable to one family may not be to another. However, children whose behaviour is constantly monitored or criticised may develop low self-esteem, which can impact on mental health. As adolescent who is parented in an authoritarian, or controlling way, may rebel and this rebellion can manifest itself in risky and unhealthy behaviours. A child whose parents are neglectful, may not have an ongoing condition such as asthma or diabetes managed as well as a parent who is attentive to the health needs of the child.

Family structure

Health outcomes for children can be influenced by the structure of the family. According to the findings from the Millennial Cohort Study (McMunn et al. 2012), children who live in a family with two parents who are in paid work have the best scores for social and emotional behaviour. The worst outcomes for children in relation to social and emotional behaviour are for those living with one parent who is not in paid work. There appears to be a link between maternal depression and poverty which has a negative influence on children's outcome. It is important to emphasise that these findings do not apply to all children and families, there will, of course, be many exceptions.

Socio-economic status

The socio-economic status of a family and the living conditions that families live in directly impacts on health. This follows a social gradient, with poor children experiencing poorer health and better-off children experiencing better health (Marmot 2020) and the greater deprivation experienced leading to higher death rates. Living in poverty can mean that conditions are 'medicalised', for instance, if parents cannot afford to change nappies frequently, a baby can develop nappy rash, this can mean that a child has a medical consultation for an avoidable reason.

Adverse Childhood Experiences

Adverse Childhood Experiences (ACEs), as the title suggests, are negative events such as bereavement and domestic abuse within families (discussed in Chapter 7). The presence of ACEs follows a social gradient, meaning that there is a higher incidence of children who experience ACEs in poorer families and the impact on children's health, especially mental health can be greater. However, it is important to point out that ACES can of course happen to all children regardless of the socio-economic status, but the impact can be mitigated by the support that is available to the family and children. The incidence or impact of ACEs on children's health can be reduced with appropriate support, those families with narrow and shallow support systems are more vulnerable. Marmot points out that ACEs 'tend to cluster' (2015, p. 119) meaning that the experiences that cause adversity in childhood such as violence in the family or a parent with addictions often occur in parallel. For many children around the world, the effects of the restrictions caused by the pandemic will have been an adverse experience.

Looked after children

In England, 'looked after children (LAC)' refers to children who have been removed from their parents, usually because of neglect or abuse, and have been moved into the care of the State. Such children have the same health issues as their peers, but their health issues can be greater because of their past experiences (DfE/DoH 2015). As well as an increase in diagnosable mental health conditions, children who are in the care of the state may have missed out on universal health services, that is health services that are available to all children, such as immunisations, thus leaving them more vulnerable to contracting avoidable infectious diseases.

Cultural and religious factors

Sometimes, cultural and religious factors can become conflated; therefore, it is important to be well-informed and be sensitive to the nuances. The culture of a family can have a profound impact on children's health. For example, Gypsy, Traveller and Roma (GTR) families tend to have poorer health outcomes, research carried out with Irish Travellers revealed that infant mortality was more than 4 times higher than in non-Traveller communities (NHS 2021). The reasons for this can be attributed to several factors. Mostly, there is reduced uptake of services because of GTR families' reluctance to access health services. However, services can be difficult to access because of the impermanence of their home addresses. An example of a religious belief that can influence health is the deeply held belief by Jehovah Witnesses that blood transfusions should not be used to sustain life.

Community

Local services and amenities within a child's community can have a direct positive or negative impact on their level of health. Poor quality housing and a lack of access to outdoor spaces can have a negative impact on children's health. Children living in deprived areas are twice as likely to be obese than those living in affluent areas (Public Health England 2018) possibly because of the environment within the community they live in. Deprived areas may not have outdoor spaces with well-maintained and safe playgrounds for children to play in and take part in enjoyable physical activity (Figure 2.3).

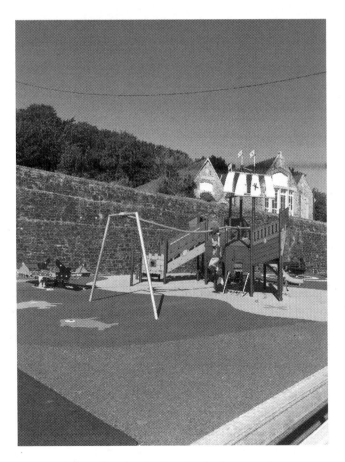

Figure 2.3 A well-maintained and safe playground.

The health of adolescents is heavily influenced by their local community, for example, banning cigarette advertising and having contraception available over the counter contribute to reducing smoking and early and unplanned pregnancy (Viner and McFarlane 2005).

Small shops in low-income areas are less likely to sell healthier foods and there is a greater number of takeaway food retailers in low-income areas (PHE 2015).

Services that meet the needs of the children and families in the local community have significant roles to play in improving children's health. Education settings in the local community can be a place of safety for some children as outlined in Chapter 5. Pre-school education and care settings, such as nurseries can play a significant role in promoting and supporting children's health (Musgrave and Payler 2021) as discussed in Chapter 4. Voluntary organisations can make a significant contribution to children's health. In the UK, Home-Start is an organisation that offers support through a network of trained volunteers to local communities. Many churches provide services for people in need, for example, food banks. Youth clubs that are well organised can provide opportunities for social interaction for young people, helping to improve their sense of wellbeing and reduce isolation, as well as being a place of safety.

Living in an area where there are effective services, both voluntary and statutory that have a whole community approach is an effective way of promoting children's health. Flying Start in Wales Flying Start is a flagship initiative launched in 2006/7 by the Welsh government to locate services in local communities to address the needs of children aged up to 4 in the most deprived areas of Wales.

Country

The number of children who die in the UK is decreasing; however, this is not the case in all countries. To illustrate this point, for every 100,000 people, there are 37.26 child deaths in the UK. In Chad, a low-income, land-locked African country, there are 1,326 child deaths.

The country that a child lives in will have a significant impact on their health. The economic wealth of a country has a direct effect impact on children's health. The poorer a country is, it is more likely that there will be a higher number of children living in poverty and fewer health services are likely to be available for children. Even if a country is rated to be high income, it is calculated that a significant number of children continue to live in poverty. For example, a high-income country such as England has a significant number of children, calculated to be 31% affected by poverty (Action for Children 2022), the impact of the pandemic has had a significant impact on the number of children who live in poverty around the world, and this is likely to increase.

In many low-income countries, children are often relied upon to contribute to their family's income to ensure their survival. It is still the case that young children work in high-risk and dangerous occupations such as mining and construction. The physical hard work as well as the risk of inhaling dust and dangerous substances can cause long-term health problems. The exploitation of children as workers in high-risk industries is similar as the situation is like the working conditions of children in the 1800s in the UK where young children were employed in factories.

In some countries where there is or has been long-term armed conflict or war, such as the Philippines, Sierra Leone and Afghanistan, young children are frequently recruited to become soldiers (UNICEF 2021b). Small children are seen to be useful as spies because they frequently escape the notice of adults; however, they are also trained to kill, often people who live in their own community. The impact of exposure to such activity at a young age is likely to leave long-lasting trauma which can affect mental health.

Ongoing conflict, natural disasters and economic needs are common reasons for people becoming refugees, often they must leave their home and country at short notice, taking minimum belongings to start perilous journeys to cross borders to see a place of refuge. The impact of becoming a refugee can cause physical privations because of hunger and lack of access to safe water, inadequate sleep and injuries. The trauma of leaving home and loved ones causes grief and other emotional responses, and in some cases, post-traumatic stress disorder and other mental health problems can develop.

The geographical location, infrastructure and political situation within countries all influence children's health. For example, areas of the world that are susceptible to drought or flooding which affects crop and food production and reduces the availability of food can be a cause of poor nutrition for all people, but especially for children. Countries that have extreme weather conditions and are also affected by political unrest or war, can have a devastating impact on food supply. The climate of a country, such as tropical countries, provides the environment where parasites and communicable diseases can proliferate, and both factors can impact negatively on children's health.

Countries that are prone to natural disasters, such as earthquakes can influence children's health. New Zealand experienced devastating earthquakes in 2010 and 2011 and research reported in the media (McCrone 2014) highlighted that the earthquakes had caused an increase in children's levels of depression and anxiety. And very worryingly, there have been reports of increased numbers of suicides in adolescents which are thought to be linked to the effects of trauma in earlier childhood following the earthquakes.

Global

The health of a country's citizens is a measure of societal success, as outlined earlier, there is disparity between how well countries can provide the environment and services that are needed to maximise the level of health of all its citizens, and this is especially the case for the youngest citizens. Efforts are being made at a global level to address the health needs of children. In many countries of the world and in some societies, significant progress has been made to elevate the status of how children are regarded across the planet. Countries with previously well-established infrastructures such as sanitation, health and education services that become war zones, leave children exposed to disease, poor nutrition and reduced health care.

The United Nations Convention on the Rights of the Child

Less than 150 years ago in the UK, many children worked in coalmines, as chimney sweeps and in factories, they were part of the workforce working in dangerous and unsanitary conditions. They did not have any workers' rights, or any rights as citizens. The work of Eglantyne Jebb, who founded the Save the Children charity in 1919, inspired the League of Nations to produce the first Declaration on the Rights of the Child in 1924. This important event highlighted the need for children to have rights to food healthcare, education and protection from exploitation. The Convention on the Rights of the Child, subsequently adopted in 1989, has been approved by all but one nation (the US) (UNICEF no date). The Convention is intended to regard children as citizens with their own independent set of rights, and sense of agency, instead of the passive recipients of adult care and charity.

However, there remain countries in the world where children's rights are denied, one example is the way that migrant children from South American countries are separated from their parents, thus denying them a right to be with their family and denying their right to health by keeping the children in conditions that impact negatively on their physical and mental health. On the US and Mexican border, migrant families who are attempting to cross into the United States illegally in search of work, or in the case of people from El Salvador because of civil strife and persecution, are arrested because of the administration's zero tolerance on illegal migration. The parents are often deported to central America, while the children are separated from their parents and there are reports of children being detained in cages (BBC 2020). The physical harm because of the unsanitary conditions and the mental harm caused by the trauma and separation from their parents are difficult to comprehend.

Many high-income countries have become home for children escaping conflict or economic disadvantage in their countries of origin; they and their families bring their health beliefs and customs with them. It is important to be aware of and respect the cultural and religious influences that can impact on children's health; however, there are some health beliefs and practices that may be unethical or illegal. One such example is the practice of Female Genital Mutilation (FGM) which is illegal in Britain; however, the practice is widespread in many areas of sub-Saharan Africa. Child marriage is a tradition in India, however, sexual intercourse when children are not ready physically or emotionally can be detrimental to health. Becoming pregnant as a young teenager has a higher chance of negative outcomes for the mother and baby.

The United Nations (UN) Sustainable Development Goals aim to improve the lives of all people in low-income countries and to 'address the global challenges we face, including those related to poverty, inequality, climate, environmental degradation, prosperity, and peace and justice' (UN 2019).

There are 17 goals that are overlapping and interrelated. Goal 3 is related to good health and wellbeing there are 13 targets that are aimed at improving health for all ages, in relation to children, there is a commitment to reduce maternal mortality, end preventable deaths in children under 5 as well as a commitment to fighting communicable diseases.

Global issues and events impacting on children's health

Climate change causing extreme weather, toxic hazards and diseases is highlighted by UNICEF as a threat to children's health because of the ways that the changes affect livelihoods and deepen poverty.

Air pollution is a risk to children's health, and this is even more significant if a school is near a main road which has heavy traffic. Children with a respiratory condition such as asthma are at greater risk of an attack if they are in an area where air is polluted Henry (2021).

Pandemics, that is, the spread of infectious across large areas of land, have affected humanity for millennia. The Covid pandemic that emerged at the end of 2019 has caused a disproportionate impact on children, for example, the loss of parental income because of unemployment and reduced family income leading to potential food poverty. There are anecdotal accounts of children demonstrating 'germophobia' because of the need for increased vigilance about handwashing.

Fitzgerald et al. (2021) assessed the impact of the pandemic in Australia, a high-income country, they state that

> the protective measures of physical distancing, self-isolation, increased awareness of hygiene practices, and school closures with distance learning has had considerable impact on children and families acutely and may have ramifications for years to come. (p. 25)

The Millennium Development Goals made 'remarkable progress' (Williams et al. 2016, p. 183). However, the Sustainable Development Goals Report (2020) outlines the negative impact of the pandemic on progress with improving health, citing the suspension of vaccination programmes and limited or no ante-natal care has increased the number of child and maternal deaths.

So far, the content of this chapter has explored some of the factors that affect and impact on children's health. Of course, the various factors cannot be separated out neatly, in reality, the factors intersect with each other.

When the factors that influence child health come together

The previous sections have attempted to unpack the factors that influence children's health and locate them into the layers that surround a child; however, all of the factors can overlap and interrelate. Please read the following case study about a small seaside town in Wales, which is drawn from a BBC news item in the summer of 2021.

Case study: life in a poor seaside town in Wales

Rhyl is a seaside town in the north of Wales. Megan is 35 and has four children.

Seren is 3, she was born early and has significant speech and language difficulties. Just before lockdown, she was being closely observed by her Health Visitor at the Flying Start centre, and she was about for a referral to a speech and language therapist. However, the Health Visitor was moved away from her usual work to work in the nearby hospital to help with the crisis, and the Flying Start nursery was only able to take the children of key workers.

Rhys and Osian are 6-year-old twins boys who have behavioural difficulties.

Dylan 13 doesn't get on with his mum's new partner, Gareth, who lives some of the time in the family home. Dylan prefers to be out of the house when Gareth is around, and recently Dylan has become friendly with a group of young men, unbeknown to him, they are grooming him to recruit him to a county line gang (there is more about county lines in Chapter 5).

The family home is cramped, there are three small bedrooms that are badly built with thin walls. The neighbours are elderly, and they get very grumpy and verbally abusive when the children are in the house. The town has few employment opportunities, so Megan is eligible for state benefits to support the children. Food is in short supply and there is limited access to supermarkets that sells affordable and nutritious produce. The local shops sell affordable bread and fizzy pop, and this forms the basis of the family diet.

Megan and Gareth's relationship is a new one, but it is becoming increasingly toxic as Gareth's alcohol consumption is getting out of hand, and he has started to hit Megan. She is becoming very depressed and has started to take anti-depressants.

Comment

Many UK seaside towns emerged about 200 years ago because sea bathing became a popular activity and people would flock to the beaches to swim in the sea, the towns grew in response to the demand. As the popularity of such towns went into decline, tourism reduced, and the towns became less affluent. Nowadays, coastal communities are some of the poorest in the UK, 'seaside towns have the highest levels of community need and poor opportunities for the people who grow up there' (Her Majesty's Government 2022, p. 4). Rhyl's geographic position means that access to areas where there are employment opportunities are less available which means that more people became poorer.

The 1970s was a time of austerity and this meant there were high levels of unemployment in the UK, thus starting a trend of 'worklessness' in families that has continued down the generations. The fabric of the town has suffered from a lack of investment during the 1980s and 1990s and this has resulted in a dilapidated and sometimes dangerous and unwelcoming environment.

As families and households became poorer, the effects of poverty and a lack of purpose partly because of unemployment resulted in many people becoming vulnerable to the availability of drugs and alcohol. Many households were using what income was available to pay for the substances they needed to feed their addictions, this resulted in money not being available to buy food for the family.

The desperation to feed addictions can lead to violent behaviour, and the target of such violence is frequently intimate partners or children. Feeding an addiction can be an all-consuming activity, which can lead to an inability to be able to care for the needs of babies and young children, consequently, many suffered from neglect. Women who become pregnant who are addicted to alcohol and drugs are more likely to have babies who are born prematurely, are 'light for dates' or are born with conditions that mean children will require on going medical attention and attendant additional needs.

Living in such circumstances can impact on people's mental health and can increase their reliance on alcohol and illegal and legal drugs to help them cope.

As 'county lines' emerged (Chapter 5), the adolescents of Rhyl became the perfect recruits to help drug dealers to provide the supply to remote areas. The involvement in young people in drug dealing, combined with violent behaviour has caused an increase in the number of crimes, and knife crime has affected the young people involved in the county lines.

The impact of the restrictions caused by the pandemic has affected the provision of services, and children like Seren, who was waiting for a speech and language therapist referral, will have potentially delayed development.

The complexities that arise from such living conditions mean that it is challenging to find effective solutions and improving living conditions in order to improve children's health requires national initiatives. In the UK, the 'Levelling up' white paper (HM Government 2022) was launched in February 2022. The aim of the Levelling Up policy put in place a raft of initiatives that will improve the quality of life and reduce poverty for people in towns like Rhyl. Implementing the aim of the 'Levelling-Up' policy will require communities to work collaboratively with local leaders who can identify the priorities that will improve the infrastructure and regenerate the area. Funding and investment will be needed to improve local transport, skills and businesses. Investing in activities specifically aimed at children and young people will help to increase their opportunities. Megan's sons would all benefit from attending planned and structured activities, such as karate classes that use up their energy and develop their physical development. Dylan could be kept occupied and potentially be safer by attending a vibrant and well-organised youth club.

Summary

This chapter has helped to set the scene for the rest of this book. It has explored some of the factors that can influence the health of babies and children from a general global perspective, many of the factors will be discussed in greater detail in other chapters. The chapter identifies the factors within the child, as well as the factors that impact on health depending on who they live with and where they live in the world. The take-away message from this chapter is that all adults have a role and responsibility to play in relation to supporting, promoting and improving children's health.

References

Action for Children (2022) How is child poverty defined in the UK? Available from https://www. actionforchildren.org.uk/blog/where-is-child-poverty-increasing-in-the-uk/#:~:text=Even%20 before%20the%20pandemic%2C%204.3,child%20poverty%20data%20in%202021, accessed 26 February 2022.

Baumrind, D. (1966) Effects of authoritative parental control on child behavior. *Child Development*. 1966; 37:887–907. doi: 10.2307/1126611

BBC News (2020) US-Mexico border: bid to reunite migrant families finds 121 more separated children, 10 November 2020. Available from https://www.bbc.co.uk/news/world-us-canada-54891974, accessed 18 August 2021.

BBC News (2021) Levelling up: the seaside town fighting violence and frustration. Available from https://www.bbc.co.uk/news/uk-58029524, accessed 18 March 2022.

Blair, M., Stewart-Brown, S., Waterson, T., and Crowther, R. (2010) Child Public Health, 2nd Ed. Oxford: OUP.

Department for Education and the Department of Health (2015) Promoting the health and well-being of looked-after children Statutory guidance for local authorities, clinical commissioning groups and NHS England. Available from https://assets.publishing.service.gov.uk/government/uploads/system/uploads/attachment_data/file/413368/Promoting_the_health_and_well-being_of_looked-after_children.pdf, accessed 23 January 2022.

Fitzgerald, D. A., Nunn, K., and Isaacs, D. (2021) Consequences of physical distancing emanating from the COVID-19 pandemic: an Australian perspective. Paediatric Respiratory Reviews 35 (September 2020): 25–30.

Global Goals for Sustainable Development (ND) 3 Good Health and Wellbeing. Available from https://www.globalgoals.org/3-good-health-and-well-being, accessed 17 August 2021.

Heckman (2022) The Economics of Human Potential: The Heckman Equation and the Heckman Curve. Available from The Heckman Equation – The Heckman Equation. https://heckmanequation.org/resource/the-heckman-curve/ , accessed 26 February 2022.

Henry, H. (2021) Focus on asthma 2: air pollution and its effects on children and young people. Nursing Children and Young People. London: Royal College of Nursing. Vol 33, No 2.

Her Majesty's Government (2022) Levelling up the United Kingdom. Available from https://assets.publishing.service.gov.uk/government/uploads/system/uploads/attachment_data/file/1052706/Levelling_Up_WP_HRES.pdf, accessed 26 February 2022.

Horn, P. (1974) *The Victorian Country Child*. Stroud: Sutton Publishing.

IHME (2022) vizhub.healthdata-org/gbd-compare. Available from https://www.healthdata.org/, accessed 12 February 2022.

Khatiwada, A., Azza Shoaibi, M. S., Neelon, B., et al. (2018) Household chaos during infancy and infant weight status at 12 months. Pediatrics Obesity 13(10): 607–613.

Marmot, M. (2010) Fair Society, Healthy Lives. The Marmot Review. Available from https://www.instituteofhealthequity.org/resources-reports/fair-society-healthy-lives-the-marmot-review

Marmot, M. (2015) The health gap. The Challenge of an Unequal World. London: Bloomsbury.

McCrone, J. (2014) Quake Stress Hurting Our Young. The Press. Available from https://www.stuff.co.nz/the-press/news/christchurch-earthquake-2011/9674021/Quake-stress-hurting-our-young, accessed 17 August 2021.

McMunn, A., Kelly, Y., Cable, N., and Bartley, M. (2012) Maternal employment and child socio-emotional behaviour in the UK: longitudinal evidence from the UK Millennium Cohort study. Journal of Epidemiology and Community Health 66(7). Available from https://jech.bmj.com/content/66/7/e19.long, accessed 26 February 2022.

NHS (2021) Improving uptake and delivery of health services to reduce health inequalities experienced by Gypsy, Roma, and Traveller people. Available from https://www.england.nhs.uk/ltphimenu/improving-access/improving-uptake-and-delivery-of-health-services-to-reduce-health-inequalities-experienced-by-gypsy-roma-and-traveller-people/, accessed 20 August 2021.

Parent and Infant Foundation (2021) Working for babies: lockdown lessons from local systems. First 1001 Days Movement. Available from https://parentinfantfoundation.org.uk/1001-days/resources/working-for-babies/, accessed 20 August 2021.

Public Health England (2015) Obesity and the environment Density of fast food outlets.

Public Health England (2018) Health matters: obesity and the food environment. Available at https://www.gov.uk/government/publications/health-matters-obesity-and-the-food-environment/health-matters-obesity-and-the-food-environment--2, accessed 29 August 2021.

Royal College of Paediatrics and Child Health (2018) Child health in 2030 in England: comparisons with other wealthy countries.

Swann, S., and Stephenson, W. (2021) Levelling Up: The Seaside Town Fighting Violence and Frustration. BBC News. Available from https://www.bbc.co.uk/news/uk-58029524, accessed 3 August 2021.

UNICEF (no date) How we protect Children's Rights. Available from https://www.unicef.org.uk/what-we-do/un-convention-child-rights/

UNICEF (2021a) The climate crisis is a child rights crisis. The Climate Crisis Is a Child Rights Crisis | UNICEF, accessed 26 February 2022.

UNICEF (2021b) Children recruited by armed forces or armed groups. Available from https://www.unicef.org/protection/children-recruited-by-armed-forces, accessed 18 March 2022.

United Nations (2020) Sustainable development goals report. Available from https://www.un.org/sustainabledevelopment/progress-report/, accessed 5 March 2022.

Viner, R., and McFarlane, A. (2005) ABC of adolescence: health promotion. British Medical Journal 330: 527–529.

Williams, B., Goenka, A., Magnus, D., and Allen, S. (2016) Child and adolescent health. In Nicholson, B., McKimm, J., and Allen, A. (Eds) *Global Health*. London: Sage.

Wilton, J., and Davies, R. (2017) Flying start evaluation: educational outcomes. Evaluation of Flying Start Using Existing Dataset. Welsh Government. Available from https://gov.wales/sites/default/files/statistics-and-research/2019-04/flying-start-evaluation-educational-outcomes.pdf, accessed 3 August 2021.

World Health Organisation (2008) Commission on the social determinants of health. Closing the gap in a generation: health equity through action on the social determinants of health. Final Report of the Commission on Social Determinants of Health. Geneva: WHO. Available from https://www.who.int/publications/i/item/WHO-IER-CSDH-08.1, accessed 18 August 2021.

https://www.denbighshire.gov.uk/en/childcare-and-parenting/flying-start.aspx

Further resources

Home-Start. A voluntary organisation offering support to families with young children. https://www.home-start.org.uk/about-us

Flying Start. A Welsh Government initiative aimed at helping families with children under 4 in areas of disadvantage. https://www.home-start.org.uk/about-us

3   Ante-natal care, screening and child health surveillance

Introduction

Over the last 100 years, but especially over the last 20 years, there has been increasing awareness of the importance of the preconception period and the influence of the ante-natal period, while the baby is in utero, that is in the womb, on the health of babies and children. This chapter focuses on some factors that can affect the unborn baby while in utero and can have long-term consequences into childhood and adulthood. Such affects may not emerge until early childhood, or perhaps even later, and can have impact on all areas of a child's development and in turn their education and wellbeing. To illustrate such an example, a case study of a child with foetal alcohol syndrome (FAS) is included. FAS is an increasing global problem and has long-term consequences on children and across the lifespan (WHO 2016).

The chapter begins with explanations about how child health screening and surveillance can make a positive contribution towards children's health. It starts with definitions of what is meant by child health and surveillance and goes on to give a brief overview of the surveillance and screening that can be carried out on babies and children during pregnancy and in early childhood.

There is some overlap between child health screening and child health promotion. Child health surveillance and screening tend to be tests and checks that are carried out to prevent disease and to detect physical and developmental abnormalities. Such interventions take place before conception, during pregnancy, after birth and in early childhood. Babies and children can be regarded as being passively involved in child health surveillance activities. In contrast, child health promotion, which is the focus of Chapter 4, involves the education of babies, children and their families in interventions and activities that are aimed at not only the prevention of health conditions but also improving the quality of health for a child in the presence of a pre-existing health condition.

What is child health surveillance and screening?

This section includes some definitions of terms used in this chapter.

Child health surveillance is a programme of secondary prevention, and it includes screening. Secondary prevention is the early detection of problems with a view to ameliorating any adverse effects (Elliman 2019, p. 201).

DOI: 10.4324/9781003255437-4

Screening can be defined as

> the systematic application of a test or inquiry to identify individuals at sufficient risk of a specific disorder to benefit from further investigation or direct preventive action, among persons who have not sought medical attention on account of symptoms of that disorder (Wald 1994, p. 76 in Elliman 2019, p. 201)

Screening tests can help to identify a problem at a very early stage and when put interventions in place can reduce the effects of the condition. The screening can be a blood test or scan, or a series of questions. In order to confirm a diagnosis, it is usual to follow up results from a screening test with more investigations.

Historical perspective to child health surveillance

Child health surveillance has its roots in midwifery (the profession that provides assistance and medical care to women before, during and after birth) and the development of ante-natal care because of concern about the number of maternal deaths in childbirth in the 1920s. The aim was to identify problems prior to labour commencing (McIntosh 2021). Midwifery and obstetrics (the branch of medicine that specialises in providing care to women during pregnancy and childbirth and afterbirth) continued to develop as specialisms over the last century. Advances in midwifery and obstetric medicine not only led to reduced maternal mortality but also to reduce neo-natal (newborn) mortality.

The role of the Health Visitor was first created in the 1860s (Adams 2012) and their focus then, as now, was on public health for children and families. Over the last 150 years, knowledge and understanding of child development has increased, and importantly, it became understood that delays or 'abnormalities' in expected levels of development for babies and young children could be a sign that there was difficulty or medical condition. As Health Visitors' role is to be involved in improving the health of babies, children and families, and they have expertise in assessing babies and children's progress with their development, their role extended to include child health surveillance.

Child health surveillance: aims and background

An overarching aim of child health surveillance is to look for developmental delay or deviations from the norm. In the 1960s, the work of Mary Sheridan (Sheridan 1960) contributed to increased knowledge and understanding of child development. Babies and children develop a range of skills: fine and gross motor skills, speech and language, social and emotional; the point at which children are expected or are likely to reach a certain level of development was referred to as a 'milestone'. The term milestone denotes that part of a journey has been achieved, and in relation to child development, milestones are behaviours or actions that a child achieves by a certain age. Sheridan's 'From birth to five years: children's developmental progress' (1973) made this knowledge accessible to professionals such as health visitors, school nurses, general practitioners, paediatricians and early childhood practitioners. This knowledge helped to create what is described as a surveillance approach to children's health and development; meaning that professionals would examine and observe babies and children to spot a condition or the lack of expertise in a child's development.

Since the start of this century, there is growing evidence of the importance of early intervention approaches to promote the long-term health of children. Approximately 20% of children experience developmental delay and identifying developmental delay or abnormalities means that interventions and or treatment can be put in place, with the aim of minimising the potential impact on the child. The surveillance approach can be described as being reactive to an existing condition or problem, in contrast, early intervention can be regarded as being proactive or preventative.

Activities used for child health surveillance

In many countries, surveillance activities are routinely carried out on newborn babies and continue to be available into childhood. There is wide variation between what is offered in countries and regions around the world. There is variation between what is offered in high-income countries (Table 3.1).

Examples of surveillance in the UK

In the UK, each baby is issued with a 'Personal Child Health Record' and the information collected about reviews is recorded in the 'Red Book' which is given to parents to keep and to take to all reviews. The Red Book also includes a record of dates when immunisations are given, as well as other health-related data and information. Babies have a series of health checks and reviews at set times which include measurement of their weight and height. Babies have a review every month until they are 6 months, reducing to every 2 months between 6 and 12 months and then once every 3 months over the age of 12 months. A further review takes place at 2 to 2 and a half years. The reviews are conducted by health professionals such as general practitioners and Health Visitors. The 2-to-2-and-a-half-year check can be conducted by a Health Visitor and a practitioner in pre-school nursery or child-minding setting if the child attends an out-of-home care and education setting. Parents are involved in all reviews, and they are asked for detailed information by completing the Ages and Stages Questionnaire to inform the 9–12 month and 2 to 2 and a half year review.

Challenges of child health surveillance

There are some challenges associated using developmental and growth charts. For example, the benchmarks that inform the norms are often based on mono-ethnic groups of children and do not take into account social and cultural factors that may impact on their development. Using the tools of surveillance also rely on the expertise of professionals taking the measurements.

There are practical considerations too, for some parents a national surveillance programme which involves multiple visits to or contacts with health professionals can present difficulties. Read the short case studies of the two babies and consider what the challenges may be.

Oliver is 9 months old, and he has started attending a nursery full time. His mum works full time and Oliver is dropped off by his mum at 7.30 in the morning and picked up at 6 pm. Oliver has two older sisters, and his dad works overseas.

Table 3.1 Summary of child health surveillance activities (content adapted from Emond 2019, also see NHS websites in further resources)

Focus	Activity	Aim of activity	Conditions that may be diagnosed
Growth monitoring	**Weight** is an indicator of growth and nutrition	To monitor weight loss in babies Failure to gain weight in childhood To monitor excessive weight gain	Feeding problems Coeliac disease, neglect obesity
	Height is a longer-term index of health and wellbeing. Often difficult to get accurate readings	Lack of growth	Growth disorder, possibly genetic or hormonal
	Head circumference can predict adult height	Enlarged head Small head	Hydrocephalus microcephaly
Physical examination	Regular examinations take place at birth, new baby visit, 6–8 week examination	To detect commonly occurring problems	Can identify problems with the heart, hips, eyes and testes
Hearing	Newborn hearing screening 9 months to 2.5 years check School entry – 4–5 years	To identify babies with permanent hearing loss To identify children who have developed hearing loss or impairment	Early identification can mean that early intervention can be put in place which can help with all round development Can be caused by head injuries, infections, glue ear
Vision	Newborn testing as part of the newborn physical examination 6–8 weeks old 1–2/2.5 years 4–5 years	To identify visual impairment of blindness	Causes of visual impairment and blindness include: Cataracts; lazy eye, squint; short or long sightedness; astigmatism and colour blindness
Development	Babies in the UK have a series of developmental reviews during the first year of life and at 2–2.5 years of age	To assess level of development. The Ages and Stages Questionnaire is completed by parents before a 9-month and 2-year development review	To identify developmental delay and possible causes, to enable early intervention

Ameenah is 9 months, her family left their country of birth and recently arrived in the UK as refugees. Ameenah and her family are living in temporary accommodation. They had a traumatic journey and are still trying to settle into England to understand the language and the different way of life on a country that is very different to the one they were familiar with. The country they left does not have a national health service as in the UK, people only sought medical services when there was a health problem.

Comment

Consider some of the challenges relating to for Oliver's and Ameenah's families. Oliver's mum has a busy schedule and is responsible for three children and her work, so she is likely to have limited time available to attend appointments. In addition, routine health services tend to be available during working hours, which is when Oliver's mum is at work, which makes it difficult for her to go to see the Health Visitor.

Ameenah's family is from another country where there is a very different approach to health. Here in the UK, there is a preventative approach to health, whereas in many countries, there is a reactive one, meaning that families only encounter health professionals when there is a problem. Adjusting to this different approach can be difficult and mean that people are reluctant to seek medical services. Ameenah's family is not familiar with the English language. As they live in temporary accommodation, they are frequently moved to different addresses, which means they may find it less easy to gain access to primary care professionals such as health visitors and general practitioners.

Oliver's and Ameenah's family situations highlight some of the practical and cultural difficulties that can be associated with accessing health professionals who carry out child health surveillance services. And of course, there are other challenges, for example, parents who have special educational needs, low levels of literacy, physical or mental health difficulties may find engaging with services difficult. Many families are not in permanent homes, for example, Gypsy, Roma, Travellers or people who move house frequently; therefore, keeping records can be less easy than for a family who remains at the same address.

Screening

Purpose of screening

In a similar way to there being greater understanding of the ways to prevent illness from occurring, this is discussed in Chapter 6, there is increased knowledge and understanding of the importance of looking for conditions that can frequently cause health problems using national screening programmes has been adopted in some countries.

Examples of screening in the UK

In the UK, as in many countries, routine ante-natal, perinatal and post-natal screening are offered to pregnant women with the aim of maximising the chances of a healthy pregnancy and the safe delivery of a healthy baby.

Ante-natal screening

Ante-natal care advances have led to treatments for many conditions that were previously untreatable; as well as treatments, there has been increased understanding of the causes of illnesses. In many countries, ante-natal screening which includes ultrasound scans and blood tests is routinely offered to identify foetal abnormalities. Identifying problematic conditions while the baby is still in utero can be beneficial to the baby and the mother or both parents. From the perspective of the baby, identifying a condition can mean that treatment can be carried out, sometimes before the baby is born; thus, preventing pain; death, the possibility of further deterioration and a chance to improve the long-term health of the baby. From the perspective of the mother or parents, the identification of a condition affecting the unborn baby can mean that they have an opportunity to decide whether they want to proceed with the pregnancy, and if not, a termination may be an option. In the event of the decision being taken to proceed with the pregnancy, knowing that the baby has a condition that may have long-term consequences for the child and the family, can present an opportunity to prepare themselves emotionally and practically.

Screening for conditions in a baby before birth appears to be a sensible intervention; however, if the findings indicate there is a problem, the decisions that need to be taken present ethical dilemmas which are complex and difficult to address.

Newborn screening

The UK newborn Screening Programme Centre defines newborn screening as a way of identifying whether a baby is at risk of carrying or being affected by genetic or congenital conditions.

In the UK, 5 days after birth all parents are offered a blood spot test for their baby, this test involves collecting a small amount of blood from a small heel prick. The blood is tested to screen for rare, but serious health conditions including sickle cell disease (an inherited blood disease); cystic fibrosis (CF), also an inherited condition which affects digestion and lungs) some metabolic conditions such as phenylketonuria (a serious condition which means that the amino acid phenylalanine cannot be broken down, leading to brain damage) and congenital hypothyroidism, a condition where babies do not produce enough of the hormone thyroid which can lead to inadequate growth and learning difficulties (National Health Service 2021).

Benefits and challenges to screening

Screening can cause anxiety for parents; however, in a study that looked at the reactions of parents whose babies were for CF, Rueegg et al. (2016) found that parents who were well-informed about the purpose and benefits of screening experienced less stress. And importantly, 88% were 'glad their child had been screened' (p. 451). Identifying the potential for or the existence of a condition that has not emerged in the newborn and not caused symptoms has significant benefits. CF can cause long-term lung damage to the extent that an organ transplant may be required to prolong life. Children with CF can be predisposed to infections which can lead to lengthy hospital admissions. Detecting the condition early can reduce the long-term impact (Figure 3.1).

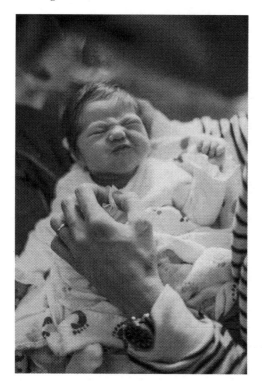

Figure 3.1 Young baby.

Source: © Brytny Com/UnsplashIMG001595.

The importance of preconception and ante-natal care for healthy babies

Ensuring the safe delivery and good health of babies starts before conception, which is described as pre-conception care.

Pre-conception care

Each child's health can be influenced by factors that are pre-determined before conception; until recently this has been an under-regarded area of children's health. There are factors that can influence the pregnancy and the child's health. These factors include lifestyle choices such as the quality of their diet, whether the mother smokes, drinks alcohol or takes illegal drugs prior to becoming pregnant (Public Health England 2018).

Ante-natal care

Care of the mother's health and management of lifestyle choices during pregnancy, that is, *ante-natal care,* can make a significant contribution to maximising babies' health and preventing conditions developing that can cause babies and children to develop additional needs during their lives. To illustrate the importance of pregnancy, the First 1001 Days Movement (Parent Infant Foundation 2022) is an alliance that works and campaigns together to promote the importance of pregnancy being regarded as part of the first 1001 days of a baby's life.

The usual period of pregnancy for babies is 40 weeks. Once conception, that is fertilisation of the egg and the start of pregnancy, has happened, the first 12 weeks is the period where the embryo develops, this is the first trimester (third) of pregnancy. After 12 weeks, during the next two-thirds of pregnancy, the foetus develops.

High-risk factors in pregnancy

The factors that can influence the pregnancy and the babies' health include lifestyle choices such as the nutritional status of the mother's diet, whether the mother smokes, drinks alcohol or takes illegal or legal drugs. The age of the mother can also be a factor that contributes to the babies' health, especially if the mother is young. Babies who have a prolonged birth, oxygen deprivation at birth, have experienced foetal distress or are born to mothers who have experienced preeclampsia (a condition that affects some pregnant women, usually during the second half of the pregnancy, from 20 weeks, or soon after their baby is delivered – NHS 2020) during pregnancy, are regarded as being at risk of developing complications.

Babies who do not have optimal conditions while in the uterus have a higher risk of being born early, that is premature (or a low gestational age), or have a low birth weight. Low birth weight babies have higher risks of brain damage and are more prone to lower cognitive scores than normal weight children, however because of the support that babies weighing less than 2.5 kg have received from neonatal services over the last 40 years, the gap has reduced (Goisis et al. 2017).

Parenting a high-risk baby

You may have heard the comment that, unlike items such as a washing machine, babies do not arrive with a booklet that gives instructions of how to feed and look after them and generally how to get the best out of them. Professional support for parenthood is part of the ante-natal care that is available to pregnant women and included in ante-natal care are practices that are aimed at maximising the chances of strong attachment bonds forming between the baby and parent(s). Becoming a parent is a time of transition and many parents can find a new baby a challenge, and some babies are more challenging than others.

Babies who are regarded as being high-risk can have immediate effects not only the babies short and long-term health but high-risk babies can present difficulties for the mother and/or parents. According to May et al., parents of infants with low birth weight have poorer perceived infant health, worse parental confidence, and they display more help-seeking behaviours. Lack of knowledge about how to interact with their high-risk infants can cause high stress and insufficient interactions with their babies for such parents (Obeidat et al. 2009). Larocque et al. have stated parental education interventions to preterm infants' parents develop parental confidence and parents' satisfaction levels (Larocque et al. 2015). In this research, by establishing a neurodevelopmental follow-up outpatient clinic, high-risk infants were followed up regularly, and families were given family training specific to the baby. As a result, it was observed that there was a decrease in the stress level of parents, and an improvement in family-infant interaction. Also, the information and support needs of the families were better fulfilled.

Foetal Alcohol Syndrome (FAS) and Foetal Alcohol Spectrum Disorders (FASD)

Pre-natal exposure to alcohol is known to result in a range of problems for babies, resulting in stillbirth and low birth weight, babies can develop FAS or foetal alcohol spectrum disorder (FASD). FASD is used as an umbrella term used to describe delays and difficulties for babies and children that are caused by alcohol consumption in pregnancy. Children can experience a range of developmental delays, which limit their participation and progress in educational and social settings. According to the British Medical Association (2016) FASD is the leading cause of non-genetic cause of disability in the Western world.

The World Health Organisation report from 2016 stated:

> The overarching principle is that "preventing, reducing and ceasing the use of alcohol and drugs during pregnancy and in the postpartum period are essential components in optimizing the health and well-being of women and their children". There is no safe level of alcohol use during pregnancy and WHO therefore recommends that health care providers should ask all pregnant women about their use of alcohol as early as possible in the pregnancy and at every antenatal visit.

The World Health Organisation is committed to addressing the problems that alcohol can cause to unborn babies, stating that 'protecting the unborn child from alcohol during pregnancy has a central place in the WHO action plan to reduce the harmful use of alcohol' (p. v). Prevention is always better than cure, but for some mothers, this is not as easy as it may sound. There are many reasons why mothers may continue to take alcohol before and during pregnancy. For example, many mothers become pregnant unintentionally and may be unaware they are pregnant for several weeks, by which time, alcohol can already have had a profound impact on the normal development of the embryo.

Identifying and diagnosing FASD

FASD is not reversible but identifying and diagnosing this condition is important because a correct diagnosis can lead to accurately targeted and effective support for children. FASD can often be misdiagnosed, and this can lead to inappropriate or unnecessary treatment and support being put in place.

Symptoms of FAS (NHS 2020)

Babies and children with FASD have distinctive facial features and may have a range of symptoms (Figure 3.2).

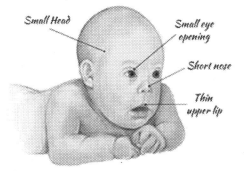

Fetal Alcohol Spectrum Disorders

Small Head

Small eye opening

Short nose

Thin upper lip

Figure 3.2 Fetal alcohol syndrome.

Source: 99healthideas.

Symptoms include the following:

- A head that's smaller than average
- Poor growth – they may be smaller than average at birth, grow slowly as they get older and be shorter than average as an adult
- Distinctive facial features – such as small eyes, a thin upper lip, and a smooth area between the nose and upper lip, though these may become less noticeable with age
- Movement and balance problems
- Learning difficulties – such as problems with thinking, speech, social skills, timekeeping, maths or memory
- Issues with attention, concentration or hyperactivity
- Problems with the liver, kidneys, heart or other organs
- Hearing and vision problems.

These problems are permanent, though early treatment and support can help limit their impact on an affected child's life.

To illustrate how FASD can impact on a child's development, please read the case study of Billy.

Case study: Billy

Billy is 8 months old, and he has recently started to attend nursery on a full-time basis. Billy's Key Person, Amrita, has been carrying out observations on him to learn more about his likes and dislikes and to identify ways to encourage his development. Amrita has become concerned about his level of development which she thinks is delayed. In addition, she is concerned about his facial appearance. She checks Billy's registration records, but his mum hasn't completed the section relating to Billy's medical history.

Amrita discusses her concerns and the lack of information in Billy's records with the senior management in the nursery. They suggest that Amrita invite Billy's mum in to have a chat about Billy's progress and development. Billy's mum accepts the invitation to attend, Amrita finds a private room to meet, and they sit down together, and Amrita explains her concerns about Billy. His mum bursts into tears and immediately explains that she discovered when Billy was born that he had FASS.

Questions

1   How would you handle this situation?
2   What sorts of questions would be appropriate to ask Billy's mum?
3   What sorts of things do you think would be helpful to Billy's mum to hear from Amrita?

Reflections

1   The feelings of guilt that a birth mother may experience can be overwhelming, and it is important that educators are supportive and sensitive, and of course not to be judgmental. Billy's mum may not have spoken about Billy having FASD previously, so it is important to listen to her, to be kind and to acknowledge her feelings.
2   The sorts of questions that are appropriate to ask include:

   •   Have you had any professional support for Billy, such as a Health Visitor? Or does Billy have ongoing treatment from a paediatrician?
   •   Have you had any information about how to help Billy?
   •   What sorts of activities does Billy like doing?

3   The sorts of things to say that Billy's mum is likely to find helpful are:

   'we can work together to learn more about FASS affects Billy'.

   'If it's ok with you, we can invite his Health Visitor to come to nursery, and she can help us to develop a care plan to put interventions in to help us to learn how to promote Billy's development'.

   'personal information relating to the health of **all** babies, children and their families is confidential'.

Of course, there are probably other things that you can think of that Amrita could say that would be helpful to Billy's mum. The case study of Billy and his mum is meant to convey the importance of being supportive and non-judgemental, not asking unnecessary questions relating to Billy and how or why he has FASS. Amrita can be professional, but warm, and convey her knowledge about Billy and his individual likes and dislikes. She can instil confidence in Billy's mum by showing that she has knowledge about FASS and demonstrating her understanding of how the staff can work together in the nursery and with other health professionals. By working together in cooperation, they can maximise Billy's potential, promote his development and minimise the impact of the symptoms on Billy.

Summary

This chapter has summarised the importance of mothers caring for their own health before and during pregnancy in order to maximise the good immediate and long-term health of their baby. However, it is important to realise that for many mothers, access to such services may be challenging. The approach to screening as a tool to identify babies who are at risk of some conditions has been summarised. The message from this chapter is to highlight the role that all professionals who work in children's services can play in child health surveillance.

References

Adams, C. The history of health visiting. Institute of Health Visiting. Available from https://ihv.org.uk/about-us/history-of-health-visiting/a-paper-by-cheryll-adams/, accessed 8 January 2022.

Blackburn, C. (2017) *Developing Inclusive Practice for Young Children with Fetal Alcohol Spectrum Disorders: A Framework of Knowledge and Understanding for the Early Childhood Workforce*. London: Routledge.

British Medical Association (2016) Alcohol and pregnancy. preventing and managing fetal alcohol spectrum disorders. Available from https://www.bma.org.uk/media/2082/fetal-alcohol-spectrum-disorders-report-feb2016.pdf, accessed 23 July 2022.

Elliman, D. (2019) Secondary prevention: principles and good practice/screening tests. In Emond, A. (Ed) *Health for All Children* (5th Ed). Oxford: Oxford University Press.

Emond, A. (2019) *Health for All Children* (5th Ed). Oxford: Oxford University Press.

Goisis, M., Ozcan, B., and Myrskyla, M. (2017) Decline in the negative association between low birth weight and cognitive ability. *Proceedings of the National Academy of Sciences*. doi: 10.1073/pnas.160554414.

Larocque, K., Heon, M., Aita, M., and Lacroix, A. (2015) Educational intervention on pre-term infants' behaviours for the promotion of parental confidence. *Infant Journal* , 11(5): 170–174. Available from https://www.infantjournal.co.uk/pdf/inf_065_ter.pdf

Martin, E. A. (Ed) (2010) *Concise Medical Dictionary* (8th Ed). Oxford: Oxford University Press.

McIntosh, T. (2021) A history of childbirth in the UK – from home, to hospital to covid 19. The Conversation. Available from a history of childbirth in the UK – from home, to hospital, to COVID-19 (theconversation.com).

National Health Service (2020) Foetal alcohol syndrome. Available from https://www.nhs.uk/conditions/foetal-alcohol-syndrome/, accessed 24 November 2021.

National Health Service (2021) Newborn blood spot test. Available from https://www.nhs.uk/conditions/baby/newborn-screening/blood-spot-test/, accessed 9 January 2022.

Obeidat, H., Bond, E. A., and Clark Callister, L. (2009) The parental experience of having an infant in the newborn intensive care unit.*The Journal of Perinatal Education*, 18(3): 23–29.

Parent Infant Foundation (2022) First 1001 days movement: evidence briefs. Available from https://parentinfantfoundation.org.uk/1001-days/resources/evidence-briefs/?fbclid=IwAR23nlS86dggQuJ8zsBTTK2XOFTLo4CongrA5olxYvfZqJVZiTwPwAI-BbA

Public Health England (2018) Making the case for preconception care: Planning and preparation for pregnancy to improve maternal and child health outcomes. Available from https://assets.publishing.service.gov.uk/government/uploads/system/uploads/attachment_data/file/729018/Making_the_case_for_preconception_care.pdf, accessed 27 February 2022.

Rueegg, C. S., Barben, J., and Hafen, G. M. (2016) Newborn screening for cystic fibrosis: the parent perspective. *Journal of Cystic Fibrosis* 15(4): 443–451.

Sheridan. M. D. (1960) *The Developmental Progress of Infants and Young Children*. London: HMSO.

Sheridan, M. D. (1973) *From Birth to Five Years: Children's Developmental Progress*. London: Routledge.

Wald, N. J. (1994) Guidance on terminology. *Journal of Medical Screening*, 1, 139–139 10.1177/096914139400100220.

World Health Organisation (2016) Prevention of harm caused by alcohol exposure in pregnancy: rapid review and case studies from member states. Available from Prevention of harm caused by alcohol exposure in pregnancy (who.int), accessed 24 November 2021.

Further resources

National Association for the Prevention of Cruelty to Children (2021) What is attachment and why is it important? NSPCC earning. Available from Attachment and child development | NSPCC Learning, accessed 27 February 2022.

National Health Service (2022a) Hearing tests for children. Available from https://www.nhs.uk/conditions/hearing-tests-children/, accessed 10 March 2022.

National Health Service (2022b) Eye tests for children. Available from https://www.nhs.uk/conditions/eye-tests-in-children/, accessed 10 March 2022.

National Health Service (2020c) Your baby's health and development review. Available from https://www.nhs.uk/conditions/baby/babys-development/height-weight-and-reviews/baby-reviews/, accessed 10 March 2022.

Open Learn Create/The Open University – Antenatal Care. A free course available at OLCreate: HEAT_ANC_ET_1.0 Antenatal Care (open.edu) part of a collection of 17 courses Health Education and Training available here OLCreate: Health Education and Training (HEAT) (open.edu).

Part II

Preventative steps that can be taken to improve the health and wellbeing of children

4 Child and adolescent health promotion

Introduction

This chapter defines what is meant by 'health promotion' which is an overlooked aspect of children's health, and the content explores some of the contemporary preventable health conditions that affect the health of babies, children and adolescents. Some of the contemporary preventable health conditions that are challenges to health are examined. The role of educators in promoting children's health and examples from practice are included.

Historical perspective: the foundations of health promotion

As infant mortality reduced during the last century, and more treatments and interventions to treat health conditions became available, there was a move away from identifying, diagnosing and treating a health condition towards looking at ways of preventing health conditions. The role of Health Visitors and the school nursing service emerged during the early part of the last century and played, and continue to do so, valuable roles in promoting children's health. However, nursery schools for young children also made significant contributions to the prevention of illness. Margaret McMillan and her sister Rachel set up a nursery school in what she described as

> a very poor, very crowded district in the south-east of London … such an environment breeds a crop of evils, the clinic we started has been crowded for 10 years with thousands of children suffering from diseases that can easily be wiped out forever.
>
> (McMillan 1919, p. 25)

The clinic that McMillan refers to is the 'minor ailments' clinic that was opened to manage the infectious diseases that were an example of the 'crop of evils' that affected the children who attended the nursery. Most of the homes did not have bathing facilities, so skin infections were common and highly communicable. In order to prevent the spread of skin diseases such as scabies, impetigo and conjunctivitis, the sisters set up 'cleansing stations' where children were bathed.

Moving to contemporary times, health promotion activities are part of the roles and responsibilities of many professionals working in children's services.

Definition of health promotion

The World Health Organisation (2018) defines health promotion as

DOI: 10.4324/9781003255437-6

Health promotion is the process of enabling people to increase control over, and to improve, their health. It moves beyond a focus on individual behaviour towards a wide range of social and environmental interventions.

This definition has informed many health promotion models, most famously, the Ottawa Charter on Health Promotion (WHO 1986), which include actions such as building healthy public policy; creating supportive environments, strengthening community actions, developing personal skills and reorienting health services. Health promotion models require individuals to learn how to promote their health by engaging with health education which is defined by the WHO (2018) as:

Health education is any combination of learning experiences designed to help individuals and communities improve their health, by increasing their knowledge or influencing their attitudes.

Health promotion and children

Health promotion in relation to children raises some considerations that are different to those when considering health promotion and adults. There are also some challenges that arise when considering health promotion in children.

Question

•   Consider the definitions of health promotion and health education above. What are the challenges and considerations when they are viewed from the child's perspective?

Comment

Your reflections may have included points such as children's:

Age – the younger children are, the less knowledge and understanding they may have about health-promoting activities, such as handwashing. As children mature and develop their knowledge, they develop greater autonomy, and they can consider factors that can influence decisions in relation to promoting their health. Promoting the health of adolescents requires careful consideration. It is less effective to have health education professionals telling adolescents to adopt healthy behaviours.

Level of development may influence children's ability to take part in health-promoting activities, for example, children with disabilities or additional needs may be limited in the amount and type of physical activity they can do. Children with cognitive impairment may have difficulty understanding some concepts relating to health promotion.

Environment and context can influence the availability of resources necessary for health promotion. This may be at national level, for example, the presence of health services. High-income countries are more likely to have an infrastructure that supports health promotion. A child's home environment influences how their health is promoted, for example, sufficient income and parental knowledge are needed to ensure that nutritional food is available.

Health promotion priorities for children around the world

Promoting children' health by focusing on ways to prevent illnesses from occurring is a global endeavour that gained momentum with the Millennium Development Goals (MDGs) which were developed by the United Nations in 2000.

Many of the health problems that emerge in adult life started in early childhood. The effects of being overweight at an early age contribute to the development of diabetes mellitus, cardiac disease and some cancers. However, these conditions can be minimised or avoided by educating children and families to adopt healthy lifestyles that promote health. The economic benefits to countries investing in improving the health of everybody is well-recognised, in addition, the benefits to individuals across the life span are compelling reasons for identifying and addressing health promotion early in life.

The ability of children to engage with health promotion activities increases with age; however, it is in the very early years that good behaviours can be shaped.

There are many conditions that affect child health across the globe for which health promotion strategies can be effective. To understand the epidemiology (that is, the cause of conditions), it can be helpful to classify health conditions into those that are 'communicable' and 'non-communicable. Figure 4.1 illustrates examples of each category and summarises prevention strategies.

Although the conditions that are summarised in Figure 4.1 are global concerns, there are conditions that are more prevalent in certain areas of the world; consequently, some of the conditions are a higher priority. In low- and middle-income countries (Figure 4.2)

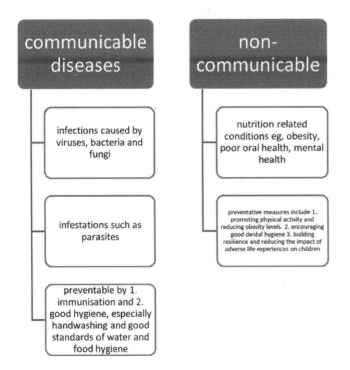

Figure 4.1 Summary of contemporary communicable and non-communicable health conditions that are preventable.

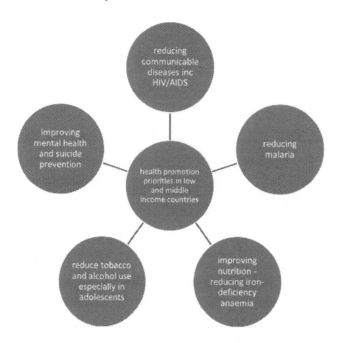

Figure 4.2 Contemporary child health priorities in low- and middle-income countries.

the priorities are driven by the incidence of communicable diseases that are threats to children's health. Many of the causes of death and illness are because of conditions such as meningitis, tetanus and pertussis (whooping cough) all of which can either be prevented or the impact reduced by implementing effective hygiene measures and by the provision of immunisations (Figure 4.3) (Williams et al. 2016).

Questions

- Consider how knowing the causes of health conditions (the epidemiology) can help to plan effective health promotion strategies.
- What are the similarities or differences between the health promotion priorities for children between low-, middle- and high-income countries?

Comment

Understanding the cause of preventable health conditions can help to identify appropriate strategies that can be implemented. Such interventions can include health education for parents and children. For example, teaching children about the importance of good handwashing techniques and providing the necessary resources to enable them to wash their hands independently at appropriate times is the single most effective way of preventing the spread of infection. You may have noticed that there are striking similarities between the priorities in Figures 4.1 and 4.2. Children and adolescents' mental health is a global concern. Suicide is a significant cause of death of young people in India and China (Williams et al.).

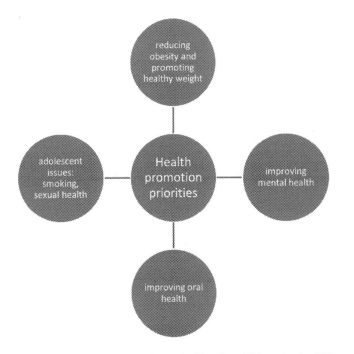

Figure 4.3 Health promotion priorities for children in the UK.

Health promotion in education settings

Children who attend school, and that is estimated to be 90% of children globally, are well placed to learn about health promotion and health education. The World Health Organisation Health Promoting School website is a source of useful information. In many countries of the world, health promotion is embedded in education curricula. For example, in Ghana, there is a well-thought-out approach to embedding health promotion in daily activities (Ministry of Education 2020). There is guidance for headteachers about their responsibility to include 10 minutes each day dedicated to delivering health messages for the whole school. The guidance is adapted to address different age groups, for younger children, the importance of road safety and hygiene is foregrounded. For older children, awareness of HIV prevention is a priority.

In the UK, the four nations have national curricula for each stage of childhood and within each curriculum, there are aims that address the health promotion needs of children. For example, the English Early Years Foundation Stage (EYFS) (Department for Education 2021) is the statutory guidance for children aged 0–5 years. Within the aims of the EYFS, there are many that link to ways that fulfilling the aims will also promote the health of young children (Musgrave 2021). However, many practitioners working in early childhood settings implementing the EYFS may not be aware of the critically important role they can make to promoting children's health. High-quality early childhood education that is implemented by highly motivated, knowledgeable and motivated practitioners can automatically make an important contribution to the health of young children (Musgrave 2019; Musgrave and Payler 2021).

In England, the Royal College of Paediatrics and Child Health (RCPCH 2017) states that effective health education embedded within a whole school approach 'can lead to improved health outcomes and improved education attainment, employability and social mobility' (p. 10). The delivery of such activities requires the efforts of all professionals involved in the education and health care of children.

Making every contact count

In the UK, the role of health promotion in schools is a major responsibility of school nurses and an aspect of their role is to 'make every contact count' which is defined as

> Making Every Contact Count (MECC) is an approach to behaviour change that utilises the millions of day-to-day interactions that organisations and individuals have with other people to support them in making positive changes to their physical and mental health and wellbeing. (Public Health England, 2016, p. 6)

The MECC approach is aimed at integrating health-promoting behaviour into every opportunity to do so, for example, taking the opportunity to point out to an individual when visiting a professional about a different matter, the importance of considering another aspect of their health.

Question

What are the benefits and disadvantages of using the MECC approach with children and young people?

You may find it useful to consider the perspectives of children, parents and professionals to consider some of the benefits and disadvantages in relation to healthy eating, as illustrated in Figure 4.4.

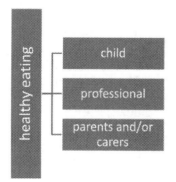

Figure 4.4 Considering healthy eating from the perspectives of the child, professional and parents.

Comment

Promoting healthy eating is a major public health priority. The negative impact of childhood obesity in childhood and into adulthood should not be underestimated (please see Chapter 9 for more about this area). However, there are many considerations to consider when attempting to integrate public health promotion messages in other encounters. You may have listed some of the points later.

Child perspective

The age and stage of development of the individual child will be critical to bear in mind. The level of understanding and vocabulary used will need to be tailored appropriately. Children who attend an appointment for something very different to what becomes a discussion about healthy eating is likely to feel offended and may feel that they are not being listened to. Children may feel there is a tension between what happens at home in relation to eating and what they are told by professionals. Children are likely to have developed their eating habits over a long period of time and making changes can be unwelcome and difficult. They may not like the healthy food options that are suggested. Lack of children's autonomy in relation to healthy eating may mean that they are unable to influence change.

Parents' and/or carers' perspective

Some parents may feel resentful about having their child counselled about their eating habits, especially when such advice is dispensed when their child is away from their care at school. Parents may have limited budgets and/or time or lack appropriate knowledge to buy and prepare food that is considered healthy. They may live in areas where it is difficult to get to retailers in order to buy affordable, healthy food. Their housing may lack food preparation facilities. Some parents may have always eaten in ways that would be regarded as 'unhealthy' but are unable or unwilling to change. On the other hand, some parents may be grateful that their child's knowledge is being increased and that healthy eating advice, if followed, is likely to improve their health.

Professionals' perspective

There are ethical aspects to delivering health promotion messages, for example, how helpful is it likely to be to a troubled 8 years old that they are overweight and should be thinking about eating a healthier diet? Professionals need to reflect on the level of skill and knowledge they possess in relation to delivering meaningful messages about healthy eating. Professionals may lack confidence in giving messages about healthy eating if they do not eat well or are overweight themselves, and this may mean they are not positive role models for children. Advice that is given in an insensitive way, may alienate children and parents.

You may have thought of other considerations about the difficulties associated with delivering meaningful advice about health promotion. By pointing out the considerations that need to be borne in mind, it is not intended to dismiss the usefulness of this approach, the intention is to caution the need for professionals to consider the feelings and individual health needs of children and their families. Such an approach has implications for planning, working in education, care and health settings using a unified multi-professional approach with good communication and relevant training at the heart of health promotion planning.

Professionals involved in child health promotion

Promoting children's health is every professional's responsibility and should be part of their role; however, it could be argued that some professionals have higher levels of knowledge and responsibility. In the UK, midwives, health visitors, practice nurses and school nurses are health professionals who are closely involved with this aspect of children's welfare. However, the role of practitioners who educate and care for pre-school children in early years settings also has a significant role. But, their role is under-researched and possibly not widely recognised, for this reason, I carried out a small-scale research project to explore what and how practitioners can promote children's health.

Research focus

I conducted a small-scale research project in a pre-school nursery in an area of high deprivation in England with the practitioners who work at the nursery (Musgrave and Payler 2021). The nursery staff wanted to become a 'healthy nursery' and to help them meet this objective they needed to work with the parents. They achieved this by:

- Practitioners communicate clearly with parents about the children's food
- Displaying the daily menus – often visually, see Figure 4.1 for how the nursery achieved this
- Taking photos of the children eating and sending them via the electronic communication system
- Providing parents with recipe cards of the dishes that children particularly enjoy
- Supporting parents to feel more confident about introducing certain food (Figure 4.5).

The approach that was developed by the participants in the research shared some aspects of the Health, Exercise, Nutrition for the Really Young (HENRY 2022) which is an approach that helps to reduce obesity in young children. However, Thornton (2019) urges caution about the HENRY programme being the reason why obesity has been reduced, instead suggesting that a significant contribution is that the practitioners used a 'whole systems approach' (p. 2), working with parents to encourage them to adopt and maintain healthy lifestyles. Similarly, participants in this research worked closely with families to do the same. Within the nursery, practitioners allocated roles and took responsibility for tasks aimed at promoting children's health; they identified opportunities to embed activities into the nursery routines, involving children and using playful approaches to teach children about healthy eating and drinking.

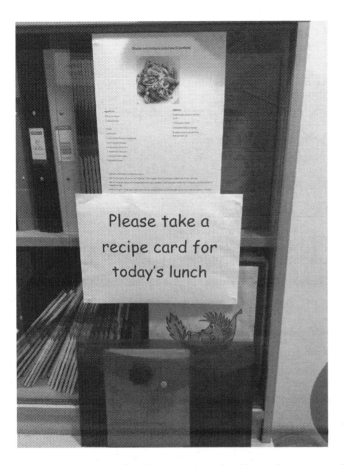

Figure 4.5 An example of how to share healthy eating menus with parents.

The participants in the research identified their role in promoting children's health; the main points are summarised in Figure 4.6.

The practitioners felt strongly that they had a responsibility to be positive role models for children. An example of how they demonstrated this was that they sat at the table at mealtimes with the children to eat and share the same food, and importantly, they chose to only drink water, like the children. As the nursery was in an area of high deprivation, it was especially important that the healthy eating and drinking approaches were relevant to the families, and that they were also realistic for busy staff and families. The resources need to be low cost and available, and the interventions adopted to promote health needed to be part of the everyday routines. Very importantly, the practitioners were keen to include the parents in the healthy eating and drinking changes, they were aiming to encourage parents to adopt some of the approaches at home. Their ability to work with parents to change habits that would promote their children's health was only possible because of the way the practitioners knew the children and the families, and also because of their ability to use sensitive approaches when working with parents.

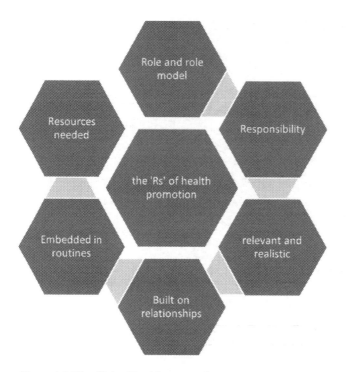

Figure 4.6 The 'Rs' of health promotion.

Health promotion for adolescents

Health behaviours relating to what can be regarded as risky behaviours often start in adolescence and can track into adult life. Evidence shows that health in adolescence can have a considerable impact on the development of adult conditions. This evidence challenges earlier notions that adolescents moving into adulthood 'grow out of' health risk behaviours and mental health problems.

According to Viner and McFarlane (2005) by far, the most effective strategy to engage adolescents is for society to adopt health promotion as a whole on behalf of adolescents, for example, by banning cigarette advertising and making emergency contraception available over the counter.

The importance of adolescents having access to professional support to promote good sexual health is highlighted by McGregor and Cannon (2016) who worked with 16–17 years olds in sexual health, they reported that building trusting relationships with adolescents is critical to help them to be willing and confident to disclose personal health information. Ross and Dryden (2021) point out the need for good communication when discussing health with adolescents, this is especially important when they may be involved in risky or illegal activities and they are concerned about getting into trouble.

Challenges and constraints to delivering effective health promotion

There are challenges and constraints that can impact on how effective health promotion can be made available to children. From a broader perspective, in a time of global austerity, a reduction in children's services can remove a conduit through which health can be promoted. For instance, in England the school nurse service has been reduced because of austerity measures, there are fewer school nurses in post and those that are in post are covering more schools and trying to reach more children. Consequently, they are likely to be spending their time with children and families who are presenting with urgent health problems.

Some families are described as being hard to reach, meaning that they are not receptive to health promotion messages. However, the factors that make such families, and in turn, their children hard to reach require examination. The factors that can influence health are examined in Chapter 2, and they are applicable to health promotion activities. For example, parents may need additional support to change aspects of routines to improve health promotion activities. Sometimes, the services may be hard to reach, for instance, working parents may find it inconvenient to access immunisation clinics that are available during their working hours.

Finding appropriate ways of delivering health-promoting messages that educate people is a challenge, and this is especially so for adolescents. Bennett (2018) reported how digital tools have proved to make health messages more accessible; however, Michel et al. (2018) in their study aimed at evaluating the use of a mental health promotion app, and were unconvinced of the effectiveness, concluding that there needs to be further work to make them more suitable and attractive to adolescents.

As highlighted earlier, some professionals not just from health but from all disciplines may not regard child health promotion as part of their role, or they may not feel they have sufficient knowledge and skills to engage with health promotion. However, we all have a responsibility to support children in promoting their health.

Summary

An aim of the chapter is to encourage you to think of how you can you work with children and families to develop relevant and sustainable approaches to health promotion. Promoting children's health must be a priority to improve the health of children for now and for their future. However, the discussion in the chapter has raised some of the tensions that may arise when taking opportunities to promote children's health. The provocations in the chapter will hopefully have given you some possible solutions to integrating health promotion activities into education and health settings.

References

Bennett, V. (2018) Breastfeeding mums can get advice through Alexa. *Nursing Children and Young People* 30(3): 14.

Blair and Barlow (2012) *Life Stages: Early Years: Annual Report of the Chief Medical Officer* [online]. London: Crown Copyright, pp. 1–13. Available from http://dera.ioe.ac.uk/18694/7/33571_2901304_CMO_All_Redacted.pdf, accessed 3 April 2017.

Department for Education (2021) Early Years Foundation Stage. Available from https://assets.publishing.service.gov.uk/government/uploads/system/uploads/attachment_data/file/974907/EYFS_framework_-_March_2021.pdf, accessed 17 July 2022.

Department of Health. (2009) *The Healthy Child Programme* [online]. London: Crown Copyright. Available from https://www.gov.uk/government/uploads/system/uploads/attachment_data/file/167998/Health_Child_Programme.pdf, accessed 21 March 2017.

Eiser, C. (1985) Changes in understanding of illness as the child grows. *Archives of Disease in Childhood* 60: 489–492.

Ghana Education Service Ministry of Education (2020) Physical and health education common core programme curriculum. Available from https://curriculum.nacca.gov.gh/wp-content/uploads/2020/02/PHYSICAL-EDUCATION-AND-HEALTH-CCP-CURRICULUM-B7-B10-DRAFT-ZERO.pdf, accessed 3 March 2022.

Health, Exercise, Nutrition for the Really Young (HENRY) https://www.henry.org.uk/about

HM Government (2018) Working together to safeguard children. Available from https://assets.publishing.service.gov.uk/government/uploads/system/uploads/attachment_data/file/779401/Working_Together_to_Safeguard-Children.pdf, accessed 1 September 2019.

McGregor, F. and Cannon, E. (2016) Assessing sexual health risk for young black and minority ethnic people. *Primary Health Care* 26(2): 18–23.

McMillan, M. (1919) *The Nursery School.* Forgotten Books. www.forgottenbooks.org.

Michel, T., Tachtler, F., Slovak, P., and Fitzpatrick, G. (2018) A review of mental health promotion apps towards their fit with media youth preferences. *EAI Endorsed Transactions on Pervasive Health and Technology* 5(17): 161419. doi:10.4108/eai.13-7-2018.161419

Musgrave, J. (2017) *Supporting Children's Health and Wellbeing.* London: Sage.

Musgrave, J. (2019) Promoting young children's health: putting it into practice. Parenta Magazine, August 2019. https://www.parenta.com/2019/08/01/promoting-young-childrens-health-putting-it-in-to-practice/

Musgrave, J. (2021) Children's health and wellbeing. In Palaiologou, I. (Ed) *The Early Years Foundation Stage: Theory and Practice*, 4th Ed. London: Sage.

Musgrave. J. and Payler, J. (2021) Proposing a model for promoting children's health in early childhood education and care settings. Children and Society. https://onlinelibrary.wiley.com/doi/full/10.1111/chso.12449

Public Health England (2016) Making every contact count (MECC): implementation guide. Available from https://assets.publishing.service.gov.uk/government/uploads/system/uploads/attachment_data/file/495087/MECC_Implementation_guide_FINAL.pdf, accessed 5 April 2018.

Public Health England (2018) Reducing unintentional injuries in and around the home among children under five years. Available from https://www.gov.uk/government/uploads/system/uploads/attachment_data/file/696646/Unintentional_injuries_under_fives_in_home.pdf, accessed 3 April 2018.

Royal College of Paediatrics and Child Health (RCPCH) (2017) The State of Child Health Report Available from https://www.rcpch.ac.uk/sites/default/files/2018-05/state_of_child_health_2017report_updated_29.05.18.pdf, accessed 17 July 2022.

Ross and Dryden (2021) How should nurses discuss substance use with young people? *Nursing Children and Young People. RCN* 33(5): 11.

Thornton, J. (2019) What's behind reduced child obesity in Leeds? *British Medical Journal News.* Analysis. Published 3 May 2019.

Underdown, A. (2007) *Young Children's Health And Wellbeing.* Maidenhead: Open University Press.

UNICEF (1996) Children in war. Available from https://www.unicef.org/sowc96/2csoldrs.htm, accessed 3 April 2018.

UNICEF (2018) Sustainable development goals. 3: good health and well-being. http://www.un.org/sustainabledevelopment/health/, accessed 5 April 2018.

Viner, R. and McFarlane, A. (2005) ABC of adolescence: health promotion. *British Medical Journal* 330: 527–529.

Williams, B., Goenka, A., Magnus, D., and Allens (2016) Child and adolescent health. In Nicholson, B., McKimm, J. and Allen, A. K. (Eds) *Global Health.* London: Sage.

World Health Organisation (1986). Ottawa charter for health promotion: first international conference on health promotion Ottawa. Available from https://www.healthpromotion.org.au/images/ottawa_charter_hp.pdf, accessed 21 November 1986.

World Health Organisation (2018) Health promotion. Available from http://www.who.int/topics/health_promotion/en/, accessed 4 April 2018.

World Health Organisation (2020) Youth violence: key facts. Available from https://www.who.int/news-room/fact-sheets/detail/youth-violence.

World Health Organisation (2022) Health promoting schools. Available from World Health Organisation. https://www.who.int/health-topics/health-promoting-schools#tab=tab_1 Accessed 5 March 2022.

Further resource

Open Learn Create/The Open University Health Education and Training – a collection of 17 free courses available from OLCreate: Health Education and Training (HEAT) (open.edu), accessed 27 February 2022.

5   Keeping children and adolescents safe

Introduction

Keeping children safe starts right from conception, a healthy ante-natal period where the developing embryo and foetus are protected from the effects of cigarettes, alcohol, drugs and trauma which helps to maximise the potential of a mother having a normal birth at full term (40 weeks). The early years of life through to adolescence can be significant times of risk because of the vulnerability of babies and children to harm. The factors and events that are risks to children's safety and cause them harm can impact on their physical and mental health. This chapter examines the unintentional and intentional risks of harm to babies and children and explores the role of adults in reducing the risk of harm to children and adolescents.

Historical perspective to contemporary times

Since Victorian times (1837–1901), there have been numerous pieces of legislation aimed at preventing harm and making children's lives safer. The novels of Charles Dickens brought attention to the plight of children who would be described as vulnerable in contemporary times. For example, Oliver Twist (Dickens 1838) was orphaned and as a 9-year-old he was sold by the workhouse staff to become an apprentice for an undertaker. Following a fight with bullies, Oliver escapes to London to find a better life. However, homeless, and hungry in London, he is taken in by Fagin, a criminal and gang leader of young boys who steal for him. While there has been almost 200 years of UK legislation to improve the lives of children, there are still children whose safety is affected by circumstances like Oliver Twist's. In some low-income countries, because of poverty, children are often needed to work to contribute to the family income. Such work frequently involves hard, physical labour. In countries where running water is not available in homes and water is scarce, young girls are frequently responsible for fetching water for the family and often must carry heavy containers over long distances. In the UK, some children are more vulnerable to harm than others, for example, children who are 'looked-after' by the State. The high-risk behaviours associated with gangs are more likely to have a negative impact on middle childhood and adolescent health. And tragically, many children are still subjected to sexual, physical and emotional abuse. Now as always, keeping children safe can be a challenging endeavour.

DOI: 10.4324/9781003255437-7

Keeping children safe

There are many actions that can be taken to keep children safe from harm, and this chapter will cover some such actions, however, it is impossible to either guarantee that we can keep every child completely safe from harm. Instead, we can consider the ways that the risk of harm to children can be minimised. The risks to children's safety are directly influenced by the child's environment within their home, as well as where they live in the world. To illustrate this point, for every 100,000 people, there are 37.26 child deaths in the UK. In Chad, a land-locked African country, for every 100,00 people, there are 1,326 child deaths, many are attributable to road traffic accidents. Some of the reasons why there is such a striking difference between the UK and the African country of Chad can be attributed to the differences between the infrastructure and services that are available in each country.

A global perspective

Children around the world are affected by economic, political, geographical and cultural factors that influence their lives and in turn, their safety. Children in war-torn countries are especially prone to exploitation. Children as young as 6, who live in countries at war, especially boys, are vulnerable to becoming soldiers. Reasons why children are increasingly recruited as soldiers include the fact that guns are available cheaply. Also, modern guns are lighter and easier to use than in the past; therefore, even young children can assemble and use guns. Refugee children who have escaped war in their countries have often had perilous journeys, sometimes on their own, which leaves them vulnerable.

Babies and young children aged 0–4 years are at greater risk of having accidents, this is partly because young children are unable to identify danger and assess risks in their environment, but also because they have small stature and can access small places. The major causes of unintentional harm and death to children is because of burns, poisoning, drowning, falls and road traffic accidents (IHME Viz Hub 2022). In adolescence, children aged 10–19, in addition to unintentional injuries, a common cause of death is suicide and homicide (RCPCH 2020).

Keeping children safe in high-income countries

In the UK, the term safeguarding is defined as the actions that must be taken in order to promote the welfare of children and protect them from harm. The aims and principles of safeguarding are outlined in the Working Together to Safeguard Children (HM Government 2018) statutory guidance. The guidance emphasises that to safeguard children, it is essential that all professionals from health, education and social care work together:

> No single practitioner can have a full picture of a child's needs and circumstances and, if children and families are to receive the right help at the right time, everyone who comes into contact with them has a role to play in identifying concerns, sharing information and taking prompt action. (p. 11)

Safeguarding can be regarded as preventative because the approaches to prevent harm should be considered in relation to every aspect of work with children. Safeguarding is broader than child protection. The consequences of not safeguarding children effectively can have negative effects on children's physical and mental health. However, there are many ethical and complex issues that impact upon how well children can be safeguarded. Consequently, it is important to increase knowledge of the influences to gain an understanding of why some children are not protected from harm. In Wales and Scotland, children are protected by law from being smacked as a means of punishment.

Safeguarding and health

In Chapter 2, living in poverty was highlighted as the single most negative impact on children's health. The factors that are associated with families who live in poverty include poor housing with the attendant risks to children's health and safety. For example, creating a safe home environment can be difficult when a family is living in housing that is not suitable for small children. Damp housing which promotes the growth of mould can provoke asthma symptoms. The home can be a dangerous place for very young children, and this is borne out by the fact that unintentional home-related injuries account for 8% of pre-school-aged children's deaths (PHE 2018). Although there is a persistent social gradient associated with unintentional home-related injuries, it is important to be mindful that young children, especially boys, are more prone to injuries in the home, their susceptibility decreases with age and increased development. Although it is also important to bear in mind that children with delayed or impaired development are more likely to continue to be at risk from injuries in the home.

Early childhood

A child's home can be the place of highest risk, and the incidence of harm to children is greater if they are living in poverty. Guidance from Public Health England (2018) states that the most common injuries sustained at home in under-fives are caused by choking, suffocation and strangulation; falls; poisoning; burns and scalds; and drowning. According to Public Health England (2019) in one area of London, in Tower Hamlets, which has high levels of deprivation, two children each week fall out of windows. This is attributable to small homes that accommodate large numbers of occupants, and the falls are often because beds are situated against windows and children can access open windows. There is a greater incidence of boys having accidents. Children are inquisitive or they may mistake items they are familiar with for similar-looking dangerous items. For instance, brightly coloured laundry capsules and air fresheners can be mistaken for confectionary.

For professionals working with children, there is legislation that ensures all are aware of the steps needed to ensure that health, education and care settings are safe for children. For example, it is mandatory for practitioners working with pre-school children to be trained in paediatric first aid. This requirement was enforced because of the increased risk of choking in young children. The risk of choking for very young children caused by seemingly harmless foods such as grapes and cherry tomatoes is a significant concern (Lumsden and Cooper 2016).

Case study: Finley

Unintentional injuries sustained at home are largely preventable by managing the child's environment; however, if a child is especially accident-prone, it is worth considering that there may be a cause from within the child as student practitioner, Jess, discovered:

Finley was having a lot of accidents resulting in minor injuries such as head bumps, grazed knees and bruises. His mum was concerned about the welfare of her child at the setting because he was injuring himself every time he was at the setting. As practitioners, we were also concerned about the well-being of Finley as he spent a lot of time upset or not involved in activities because of his injuries. For example, we had to sit Finley out with a cold compress or administer first aid. We were also disrupting his play a lot when we pre-empted accidents.

When we spoke with Finley's mum, she explained that she was really stressed. We discussed Finley's accidents and assured mum we were doing everything we could to try and stop them from happening. She said his 2-year check was coming up and she would ask the health visitor, but she felt in the meantime she wanted to withdraw Finley from the setting because the number of accidents he was having couldn't be good for him. After more discussion, I raised the idea of an eye and hearing test for Finley just to ensure there wasn't a medical reason for the accidents, such as, loss of sight or hearing. Finley's mum agreed she would get the tests done and report back to us. Finley went for an eye test, and it was found that he was severely visually impaired in one eye. When Finley's mum reported this to us, we immediately adapted certain aspects of our practice, in collaboration with Finley's parents, to make the environment more suitable for him. This included but was not restricted to providing fluorescent name tags so Finley could find his name with more ease, putting florescent tape around door frames, edges of furniture and steps where it was common for Finley to have accidents and ensuring when we spoke to Finley, we communicated e.g., made eye contact with his 'good eye'. We saw significant improvements in Finley's quality of experience at the setting and the parents were very grateful we had worked so closely with them in ensuring we got the environment right for Finley.

Question

- How did Jess's critical thinking about Finley help to improve his health and well-being?

Comment

When a child is experiencing unintentional injuries, the consequences for the child can be profound as highlighted in the case study above. However, unintentional injuries can be damaging to relationships, raising suspicion about the capability of all who are involved in children's care to keep them safe. In this case study, Jess describes how she was able to work with Finley's mum to help her consider alternative explanations as to why Finley was experiencing so many injuries. She then explains how she assessed the suitability of the environment for Finley and identified how adaptations could be made which would keep Finley safer. Jess's critical thinking, that is, using her knowledge and understanding helped her to observe, assess and evaluate Finley's environment, and by working with his mum and colleagues, she was able to lead on making his environment safer for him.

Middle childhood

As children reach middle childhood, around 8–12 years of age, there is an increase in the levels of independence and a change in the level of supervision required to keep children safe from harm. For most of the last century, children mostly played outdoors in the streets and other public areas. This tradition means that children benefitted from high levels of physical activity and developed independence and social skills. In the 1990s, following a series of highly publicised child abductions and murders, public opinion, influenced by the media, seemed to change and the tradition of children playing outdoors in public places reduced. It is important to bear in mind that children have always been a target and child exploitation and murder is not a new phenomenon. However, increased media attention fuelled concern amongst parents. As well as children having opportunities for outdoor play curtailed, technological developments meant that other entertainment options were available, such as electronic games. Such games appeared to captivate children's imaginations and in the climate of fear provoked by the danger that children were perceived to be in by playing in public places, many parents were relieved that the games could be used as so-called 'electronic babysitters'. More than a quarter of a century on from the introduction of electronic games, babies and very young children are frequently given phones and iPads as ways of entertaining them, so the problems associated with reduced physical activity are now affecting children in their first year of life. With increased access to electronic ways of communicating with the world, the opportunities for children to become vulnerable to exploitation have also increased; such exposure can impact upon mental and physical health.

Keeping adolescents safe

The physiological changes to brain architecture caused by changes to synapses during puberty and adolescence affect children's ability to read emotions and assess risk. As children reach adolescence, their lifestyle means they have greater autonomy, such as walking to school independently, socialising with peers without adult supervision and this naturally means that they are potentially at greater risk of harm. This period of late childhood is associated with an increase in risk-associated behaviours such as experimentation with smoking, sex, alcohol and illegal drugs. The emotional impact of factors caused by nutrition such as obesity, anorexia and eating disorders are keenly felt at this age.

Adolescence is a stage of significant inner turmoil, the addition of adverse life experiences, such as family break-up, can be another unwelcome addition for young people making the transition from childhood to adulthood even more challenging, which increase the chance of them engaging with risk-taking behaviours which can impact on their health. The following case study illustrates the profound impact that an unplanned pregnancy had on a 17-year-old Ghanian schoolgirl.

Case study: Jane

By Joyceline Alla-Mensah

Jane is a 17-year-old girl from the Western region of Ghana. She is a second-year, boarding student in a Senior High School which is several kilometres from her hometown.

She aspires to be a mechanical engineer and has an undiagnosed learning difficulty that affects her learning and performance in class. She got pregnant at 16 years and knowing that teenage pregnancy is frowned upon, she hid it from her family, teachers and school authorities, until it was later discovered by her peers who informed her housemistress. The school authorities called for a meeting with her parents, and they were informed that Jane cannot be accommodated at the residential facility and would be made a day student. It was explained that the boarding facility was not safe for her and the baby and living at home might enable her to receive more support from the parents. Considering the impracticality of continuing as a day student, the parents sought a transfer to a school in her hometown. She was rejected, with no explanation and Jane's family suspected that it was due to her pregnancy. Jane had no option but to drop out.

Throughout her pregnancy, her friends disconnected from her, as their parents perceived her to be a negative influence on them. While she was keen to continue learning at home, she did not have any learning support and struggled to comprehend the textbooks. Six months after giving birth, Jane re-enrolled in the school in her community. She was told she had to repeat the previous academic year to catch up with lessons missed. In class, she was constantly stigmatised by her teachers and schoolmates and not being able to contain the stigma, bullying and the humiliation, she dropped out. While Jane feared that her dream of becoming an engineer had ended, her parents helped her to enrol in an informal apprenticeship training to acquire skills in the automotive trade. While Jane can achieve her aspiration through this alternative route, she has been denied the opportunity to complete her secondary education and obtain the certification needed to pursue higher education.

Comment

Ghana recently introduced a policy for the prevention of pregnancy among schoolgirls and facilitation of re-entry into school after childbirth. The policy stipulates that pregnant girls need to remain in school until they are due to deliver. The case study underscores the importance of creating an inclusive school environment where pregnant schoolgirls are not stigmatised and discriminated against. In highlighting the relevance of an inclusive environment, a case is also made for strengthening mechanisms for reporting abuses. However, Jane's experience highlights that there is a need for education about safe sex and avoiding pregnancy.

Adolescents with difficult circumstances will be especially vulnerable at this stage; Jane's learning difficulty made her vulnerable to becoming pregnant. In the UK, 'looked after children', a term used to describe children who are looked after by the state rather than in a traditional family unit, are known to have poorer health outcomes (NICE 2021). If a child is frequently moving between foster parents or children's homes, with several professionals responsible for maintaining their health, there is a need to ensure that effective inter-professional working practices and policies are in place to keep track of children's health needs.

There is often a strong desire by most adolescents to be part of a social group with a strong sense of belonging to identifying with such groups, this can make some children vulnerable to being recruited to gangs. According to the World Health Organisation (2020), youth violence is a global public health problem, the impact of which can result in death or in long-term physical and emotional consequences. In the UK, Children from the age of 12, but most commonly from the age of 14–17 are targeted to become involved in county line activity. County lines are 'gangs and organised criminal networks involved in exporting illegal drugs … using dedicated phones to take orders for drugs' (HM Government 2018). Recruited children are enticed into distributing and selling drugs by 'gifts' of drugs and money (Rosengarten 2021). As well as being responsible for moving and storing drugs, they are subjected to coercion, intimidation and violence, including sexual violence and the use of weapons.

Some children find it difficult to make the transition and many children who find it difficult to conform to the norms of being at school are frequently excluded from attending school. Removing children from school does not solve the 'problem' of an adolescent finding it difficult to fit in and be part of a school community, it simply transplants the 'problem' into other areas of society. Recent reports suggest that children who become involved in adolescent gangs are more likely to have been excluded from school. As children who are victims or perpetrators of knife crime are more likely to be involved in adolescent gangs, this suggests that examining the reasons why some children feel excluded from the society of their secondary school could be a helpful step to reducing the culture of gangs and knife crime.

Modern slavery and human trafficking

It is estimated that globally, 1 in 4 victims of modern slavery are children (Unseen 2020). Modern slavery is defined by the British government as 'the recruitment, movement, harbouring or receiving of children, women or men through the use of force, coercion, abuse of vulnerability, deception or other means for the purpose of exploitation'. In the UK, there are a significant number of children who become pawns of organised crime groups earning vast amounts of money for these groups. It is anticipated that the pandemic will have increased the number of people who become enslaved because of increasing poverty. Children are recruited into modern slavery for the sex trade, with children as young as 14 working as prostitutes. The following case study illustrates how a child in the UK can face harm and the potential impact on her physical and mental health.

Case study: Sky

Sky is 15 and has never lived with her parents, her mother lived 200 miles away with a man who didn't want the complication of having a baby living with him and Sky's mum, both were addicted to drugs and alcohol. As is often the case for many children whose birth parents cannot care for them, she was passed over to Sky's mum's parents, who became her kinship carers and they brought her up for the first 5 years of her life. Her grandparents struggled to look after Sky, she had learning difficulties because of the effects of foetal alcohol syndrome which she developed because of her mother's addiction to alcohol when she was pregnant with Sky. The situation became particularly bad when Sky's behaviour deteriorated after her grandfather had a stroke and he could no longer contribute to caring for Sky. The pressure of having to look after Sky's grandfather following the stroke along with him no longer playing an active role in caring for her meant that her grandmother could no longer cope, and she had to put Sky into the care of the State and become a 'looked after' child.

Sky's life continued to be tumultuous, she had vivid memories of the few times that she had met her mum, but the visits caused Sky so much distress when her mum left, that her grandparents got to the stage where they had to stop them from happening. Sky had already felt rejected by her parents and what she saw as rejection by her grandparents tipped her behaviour over to the point where she was almost un-manageable, she illustrated the point that the children who behave in the most un-lovable ways are those who are most in need of love. Sky went to live with several foster families but none of them was able to offer her a long-term home, and Sky lived in a children's home from the age of 8.

As Sky entered adolescence and turned 13, the home that she lived in became a target for a local organised crime group, one of the men befriended Sky, he offered her sweets, clothes and money, but most of all he listened to her, spent time with her and gave the hugs and cuddles that she craved, telling her that she was his best friend. When he suggested that Sky would be an even better friend if she was willing to meet some of his friends and allow them 'to play with her', she willingly did so, and Sky was delighted to have attention from so many people and to receive money. However, when Sky turns 16, she is no longer needed by the gang and her 'friend' turns his attention away from her and moves on to other younger girls. Sky became angry and hurt and once again, she felt as if she had been rejected. Sky soon finds herself the target of another gang that run a brothel, which is based in a large old house which is run down and filthy. In return for sex services for the clients who visit the brothel, she is given somewhere to live, a couple of meals a day, usually takeaway or convenience food, as well as drugs and alcohol that help her to feel better. Living in the brothel has mixed benefits for Sky. On the one hand, she has company because she is living in a house and there are other girls her age, and even though there are arguments and rivalries, she feels better than if she was living alone on the street. And more than anything she knows that she can get regular supplies of drugs and alcohol. However, she is becoming scared of some of the clients who are physically abusive, and she is expected to have sex with as many as 12 clients each day. But she is trapped by the gang and knows that she cannot escape.

Critical questions

1   How has the adversity that Sky experienced contributed to her becoming involved in the sex industry?
2   What are the risks to Sky's physical and mental health?

Comment

There is no typical victim of modern slavery, it tends to be people who are regarded as vulnerable, such as those who exist on the margins of society who are more likely to be exploited and become a victim of modern slavery. Sky was especially vulnerable because the effects of having foetal alcohol syndrome will have affected all areas of her devel-opment. For example, her cognitive impairment may have impacted on her ability to engage with her education. The behavioural problems that she developed because of the adverse early life have been a series of rejection and broken relationships which meant she was vulnerable to the attention given to her by the paedophile gang.

Sky's living environment is a risk to her health and safety. There are significant risks to her physical health because of the unsanitary conditions in the house. As she is a captive of the gang, she is not allowed out of the house, so she has limited physical activity outdoors. While Sky generally has enough to eat, her diet is inadequate, and she is probably under nourished. Her physical and mental health will be affected by the increasing addiction to alcohol and drugs. Sky is at risk of contracting a sexually transmissible disease as well as being at risk of becoming pregnant. People who are kept in slavery will not have access to appropriate health care, or dental care. Sky's fears about physical violence, her growing addictions and the legacy of her early experiences are all factors that contribute to poor mental health.

The role of education settings in keeping children safe

Early childhood and school settings can be a place of safety or a place where children can experience harm. There have been cases of practitioners who have abused babies and children within their care (Birmingham Safeguarding Children Partnership 2022) and children frequently experience bullying in schools. The potential sources of harm to children in education settings are numerous, and much is done to ensure that the risk of harm to children in education settings is identified and acted upon. (Department for Education 2021).

On the other hand, education settings for babies, children and adolescents make a significant contribution to their safety. It is a statutory requirement that early years pre-school settings, schools and colleges ensure that the environment is maintained in a way that ensures a safe environment and minimises risks to children. In addition, professionals are responsible for the safeguarding of babies and young children and are alert to the signs of risky behaviour and abuse. Health promotion (Chapter 4) is embedded in the curricula and teaching children about the consequences of risky behaviour can minimise risk and subsequent harm.

The restrictions caused by the pandemic have revealed the importance of education settings in reducing harm to children. The closure of pre-school settings and schools meant that children spent more time at home. In England, research by the National Society for the Prevention of Cruelty to Children (NSPCC) (Romanou and Belton 2020) explored the risk to children's safety due to the conditions created by the COVID-19 pandemic in the UK. They found that the risk of harm to children is higher when families and carers experience stress, and the restrictions were a cause of stress to many families. During the period of school closures, children were more vulnerable to abuse both online and within the home. Changes to the way that protective services were provided to children and families during the pandemic left children more vulnerable to harm. The findings indicate that attending education settings can be a place of safety for many children.

In December 2021, a media report (Savage 2021) published findings from Local Authorities (who are responsible for monitoring and reporting children's attendance at school) in England that there were tens of thousands of children who were not attending school and had disappeared from official view. Many of the missing children are known to have mental health difficulties, special educational needs or disabilities and are therefore deemed to be vulnerable, thus leaving them more likely to become targets for abuse and harm.

Summary

This chapter has highlighted that many of the threats to children's safety that used to exist in the past remain threats in contemporary times. It is important that children are taught about their role in reducing vulnerabilities that can make them more susceptible to being the target of others who want to harm children. However, it is important that this approached in ways that do not create anxiety and unnecessary concern, but this can be a difficult balance to get right. It is the responsibility of all adults in children's lives to be aware of their role in keeping children safe, or as safe as possible. There is a critical role by all professionals to be aware of how children's services can keep them safe. In particular, education settings can be a place of refuge from harm for many children, and there is a critical role for all educators to be aware of how they can contribute to preventing harm to children.

References

Birmingham Safeguarding Children Partnership (2022) Learning lessons from serious cases.

Department for Education (2021) Keeping children safe in education: statutory guidance for schools and colleges. Available from https://assets.publishing.service.gov.uk/government/uploads/system/uploads/attachment_data/file/1021914/KCSIE_2021_September_guidance.pdf, accessed 10 March 2022.

Dickens, C. (1838). *Oliver Twist*. London: Simon and Shuster.

IHME (2022) vizhub.healthdata-org/gbd-compare. Available from https://www.healthdata.org/, accessed 12 February 2022.

Lumsden, A. J., and Cooper, J. G. (2016) The choking hazard of grapes: a plea for awareness. *Archives of Disease in Childhood*. doi:10.1136/archdischild–2016311750.

National Institute for Health and Care Excellence (2021) New draft guidance aims to achieve fairer outcomes for looked-after children and young people. Available from https://www.nice.org.uk/news/article/new-draft-guidance-aims-to-achieve-fairer-outcomes-for-looked-after-children-and-young-people, accessed 5 March 2022.

Public Health England (2018) educing unintentional injuries in and around the home among children under five years.

Romanou, E., and Belton, E. (2020) Isolated and struggling: social isolation and the risk of child maltreatment, in lockdown and beyond. NSPCC Evidence team. June 2020. Available from Isolated and struggling: social isolation and the risk of child maltreatment, in lockdown and beyond (nspcc.org.uk), accessed 18 February 2022.

Rosengarten, L. (2018) County lines crime: what is a nurse's role in safeguarding children? *Nursing Children and Young People*. London: Royal College of Nursing.

Royal College of Paediatrics and Child Health (2020) *State of Child Health*. London: RCPCH. Available from stateofchildhealth.rcpch.ac.uk.

Royal Society for the Prevention of Accidents (2021) Accidents to children. Available from https://www.rospa.com/home-safety/advice/accidents-to-children#why, accessed 1 August 2021.

Savage, M. (2021) Hunt launched to find 'ghost children' missing from schools in England. Observer Newspaper. Sunday 12 October 2021. Available from Hunt launched to find 'ghost children' missing from schools in England | Child protection | The Guardian. Accessed 18 February 2022.

Unseen (2020) Modern slavery facts and figures. Available from Facts & figures - Unseen (unseenuk.org). Accessed 12 February 2022. https://www.theguardian.com/society/2021/dec/12/hunt-launched-to-find-ghost-children-missing-from-schools-in-england

Part III

Supporting children with health conditions

6 Communicable, infectious and parasitic conditions

Introduction

Communicable diseases and parasites are a significant cause of poor health globally. The global pandemic that started in spring of 2020 illustrated the point that infectious diseases do not recognise borders (Davies 2019, p. 1). In a world where air travel is common and people cross country borders, the transmission of infection is relatively easy and therefore, the challenge to control infection is more difficult. Infection prevention and control is an important part of achieving universal health coverage for all, but globally this aspect of health does not receive adequate attention. According to Storr, Kilpatrick, Allegranzi and Syed, 'hundreds of millions of people are affected by avoidable infections in health care setting' (2016, p. 40). The reasons why infection affects so many people include lack of adequate handwashing facilities and insufficient levels of training and motivation amongst staff. In relation to children, the control of infection raises many issues. Children in pre-school and school settings come together in large numbers and are in close proximity with each other, ideal are conditions that help to spread infections. A child's ability to be aware of what their responsibilities are in relation to preventing infection relies partly on their age and stage of development. There are other factors that impact on how much children are protected against infection, such as where they live in the world; their parents' or carers' health beliefs and choices; the level of knowledge of educators and other professionals as well as the child's level of vulnerability to infection. In a similar way, parasites can impact on health and wellbeing, causing symptoms that can range from being regarded as minor irritations, or on the other hand, the symptoms of some parasites can be severe and potentially life-threatening.

The pandemic has focused our attention on the importance of preventing infection, however many of the precautions that were advised, such as regular handwashing, care with bodily fluids and taking up the offer of immunisations is exactly what we should be doing all of the time (Musgrave 2020).

This chapter defines some of the terms associated with communicable diseases, as well as some of the contemporary communicable conditions that affect children from a global perspective. It will also explain the ways that the spread of infection can be prevented, and it explores some of the ways that communicable diseases and parasites can impact on children's health. In particular, the chapter explores some of the ethical tensions that can arise because of parental choice, particularly in relation to immunising their children against infectious diseases, and it will explore some of the factors that can influence their choices in relation to preventing infection in children.

DOI: 10.4324/9781003255437-9

Definition, causes and transmission of infection

Infections are caused by micro-organisms, which can be defined as living organisms that are not visible to the naked eye. This fact is of course one of the reasons why infections can spread with relative ease, it is simply because the micro-organisms cannot be seen, therefore, viruses, bacteria and fungi, which cause infections can enter the body in several ways without detection.

Infections can be spread and enter the body in the following ways:

Direct contact – *close physical contact.*
Vertical transmission – *from infected mother to her baby during pregnancy or birth or via breastmilk.*
Inhalation – *breathing germs into the lungs.*
Inoculation – *entering the body via the skin.*
Consumption (or ingestion) – *swallowing contaminated food or water, or via faeces transported on the hands, for example, when hands are unwashed following defaecation.*
Indirect contact – *touching a contaminated surface and then transferring germs to the eyes, nose, mouth or into an open wound.*
Vehicles or vectors – *via animals or insects.*

As babies and young children require support with their physical needs, it is obvious that the adults who work with them are going to come into close contact with bodily fluids. Young children need to be taught self-care from an early age so they learn how to manage bodily functions which can spread disease.

Historical perspective

Throughout history, infectious diseases have caused epidemics that have killed millions of people around the world. In 1665, in London, England, the bubonic plague was spread by fleas in rats, and it is estimated that about 100,000 people died (National Archives website). The plague's spread was halted when the following year, in 1666, the Fire of London helped to destroy the rats who transmitted the plague.

A vital step in understanding how some infectious diseases could be prevented was because of the work of Edward Jenner in 1796. Jenner noticed that some milkmaids did not succumb to smallpox because they became infected with the less deadly cowpox which protected them (Davies 2019). Jenner coined the term vaccination and his findings eventually resulted in the World Health Organisation declaring in 1980 (WHO 2019) that smallpox had been eradicated globally, thus a communicable disease which had previously scarred and killed many people had been removed.

Another example of how a communicable disease can result in an epidemic, or in this case a worldwide outbreak, that is pandemic, was caused by an influenza epidemic in 1918 which killed more people than had been killed in the First World War.

In the 1895 edition of 'The Family Physician' (Cassell and Company), it is stated that 'there is no more terrible disease than diphtheria … one of the most prominent diseases of infantile life' (p. 54). This is because diphtheria affects the mucous membranes in the throat and 'covers them with a tough and leathery membrane' (ibid) which leads to obstruction of the airway, accompanying difficulty in breathing which can lead to suffocation and death. With increased understanding about how infectious diseases are caused and better treatments were developed, the threats caused by infectious diseases started to diminish. As the impact of such infections reduces, this can mean that people forget how lethal they were, and in turn this can bring complacency about the dangers.

Global perspective of communicable diseases

In many low-income countries, infectious diseases, some of which are regarded as belonging to the past in higher income countries continue to be a threat to health and life. Cholera outbreaks have caused many deaths throughout history and continue to do so in contemporary times.

Contemporary communicable conditions

The focus on universal health coverage for all is especially relevant to communicable diseases. Infectious diseases affect hundreds of millions of people each around the world with most cases being in low-income countries where the basic requirements of sanitation are not established, and this has resulted in a global increase in the number of cases of infectious diseases.

As mentioned above, a lack of safe water and sanitation are major causes of high infection rates, but when civil unrest or natural disasters happen, spread can happen rapidly. The Chief Medical Officer Report (Davies 2019) gives the example of the two cholera outbreaks in Yemen, a country that has endured civil war, to highlight how a combination of unclean water for 16 million of the 28 million population, combined with no public services have meant that over a million people and it is estimated that 2,500 people have been killed because of cholera.

Tuberculosis kills 1.6 million people globally and because the infection requires up to 6 months which is a lengthy period to complete the treatment regime, this is one of the reasons why it is especially difficult to reduce the number of cases. Unaccompanied asylum-seeking children are especially at risk.

Sepsis 'is a global killer and can have lifelong consequences for those who survive it' (Priday 2019, p. 12). Sepsis is the body's response to infection and can cause organ failure, damage and death. Sepsis is very difficult to diagnose, especially in children. Survival rates are improved if antibiotics are given within an hour of diagnosis; however, this is not always achievable if there is a delay because of availability or access to treatment. See UK Sepsis Trust for more information.

People are especially vulnerable to infections and parasites when the living conditions are poor, when there is no clean water available, a lack of public services and poor sanitation all add to a toxic combination that enables the micro-organisms that cause infection to spread quickly. This highlights some of the difficulties that can become barriers to preventing and controlling the spread of infection.

Prevention of infection

Before houses were built with plumbing that provided running water and flushing toilets, and before the underground sewerage system was invented, poor sanitation led to frequent incidents of infectious diseases, often with fatal consequences for children. In contemporary times, high- and middle-income countries tend to have the infrastructure which supports good sanitation and this in turn reduces the risk of infectious diseases. However, in low-income countries, a lack of infrastructure means there is a higher level of infectious diseases, which remain a threat to health.

Breastfeeding is known to be a way of preventing infection in babies. Fewer mothers breastfeed their babies in high-income countries, therefore babies miss out on the protection from infection that is available from the mother in breastmilk. The impact of protection from infection via breastmilk is illustrated by Parashar et al. (2015) who note that there is an increased number of babies admitted with gastroenteritis caused by rotavirus, and the number of hospital admissions was found to be higher in industrialised countries.

The main ways of preventing infection according to Public Health England (2014) include:

1   High standards of personal hygiene, particularly handwashing
2   Maintaining a clean environment
3   Routine immunisations.

These ways will be explored in more depth in the following sections.

High standards of personal hygiene and handwashing

Hand hygiene

The Royal College of Nursing (2016) states that 'regular and effective hand hygiene is the single-most important thing you can do to protect yourself and others from infection. Their guidance emphasises that hand hygiene involves hand washing and hand drying and goes on to remind us that the process of drying is as important as the process of washing.

This is a globally accepted fact to the extent that UNICEF promotes ways for people to develop good handwashing techniques through health education and promotion events, such as 'Handwashing Day' (UNICEF 2019).

Teaching children to develop good hygiene can be problematic, and the following sections consider some of the factors that may impact upon how children take care of their personal hygiene, including handwashing.

Age and stage of development

How much children can do to prevent the spread of infection partly depends on their age and stage of development. Children who have special educational needs may have limited understanding of how infections and parasites are spread and may require support beyond the time that it would be expected they could start to take greater responsibility for their self-care. Children with complex medical needs are also more likely to require support with self-care.

EARLY CHILDHOOD

Encouraging children to learn about the importance of health-promoting behaviours in relation to preventing the spread of infection is important right from the earliest time of life. Teaching children the importance of managing their own bodily fluids is a powerful way of containing the micro-organisms that spread infections.

MIDDLE CHILDHOOD

In this age group, children can be responsible for much of their personal hygiene and the need for prompting children to comply with good standards of hygiene may reduce. However, there is no room for complacency and reminding children of the need to wash their hands properly can help to reinforce the messages.

ADOLESCENCE

The experimentation with new behaviours in adolescence can extend to sexual behaviours; therefore, it is important that sex education includes awareness of infections that are transmitted via sexual intercourse. How and when this is done depends on where and how health promotion information is accessed. In many countries, such information is provided as part of the curriculum and as part of a school health service.

Starting university can be a time when young people are especially vulnerable to infectious diseases and many universities have implemented health education programmes to help avoid the spread of infections such as meningitis. Chlamydia is especially prevalent in university students and preventing the spread of this sexually transmitted disease is an important focus of health education.

Cultural perspectives

Culture can influence beliefs about the causes of how infectious diseases spread. An Ebola outbreak started in the summer of 2018 in the African country of the Democratic Republic of Congo resulted in the death of hundreds of people. Ebola is caused by a virus, which is spread by close physical contact and is fatal in 90% of those who become infected with the disease. However, in a survey carried out in Congo by the Lancet Infectious Diseases Journal (Vinck 2019), a quarter of respondents claimed that Ebola does not exist. Instead, it is believed that doctors kill healthy people and sell their body parts to devil worshippers. Another theory was that Ebola is part of a conspiracy theory made up by people in the west. Where such beliefs exist, it is difficult to educate people about the causes of infection, thus implementing strategies that can promote understanding of how to prevent the spread is difficult. Such difficulty is compounded by the associated stigma which increases fear and stifles those who understand the nature of infectious diseases from having influence to make positive changes.

The imperative for preventing the spread of infection

There are compelling drivers for preventing the spread of infection. There are economic drivers because preventing infection helps to reduce the amount of funding on health services. Davies (2019) highlights that for every dollar spent on immunisations, $16 dollars are saved in treating the effects of infection.

From an individual point of view, avoiding infections means that a child is likely to have an increased sense of wellbeing, they are more likely to engage with activities and be able to concentrate on their learning, and this in turn, can mean they are more likely to meet their potential. Communicable disease, even the common cold, which if often considered a 'mild' illness can make people feel unwell and can impact on children's wellbeing and educational attainment

> Even though illnesses that are relatively minor and of short duration may not necessitate visits to the doctor, it seems plausible that children who experience minor illnesses on a recurring basis may be at an increased risk for poor developmental outcomes. (Kolak et al. 2013, p. 1234)

Dehydration and lack of appetite can be other effects of an infection. The symptoms of such infections can impact profoundly on young children especially if they do not understand why they feel unwell and especially if they do not have the vocabulary to express their feelings. Other consequences of infectious disease can include diarrhoea causing fluid loss which may need the replacement of electrolytes and fluid replacement. Dehydration is the biggest cause of death in children following diarrhoea and vomiting, especially in low-income countries. And although medication can be given to stop diarrhoea, there are side effects from the reduction in peristalsis which can lead to constipation. Other side-effects can include sepsis resulting in long-term damage and potentially in death.

As well as the more obvious effects of the symptoms of infection, there are other reasons why avoidance is beneficial, an interesting example emerged in my health promotion research where practitioners reported how an infection impacted upon healthy eating. This was because many of the children had been diagnosed with hand, foot and mouth, an infection that spreads with ease amongst humans in close proximity to each other. The ulcers that appear in the mouth which is a typical symptom of the disease can be very painful. This can affect the children's ability to eat and drink because it is painful. The pain can also mean that children dribble, which makes transmission of the disease even easier (Musgrave and Payler 2021).

Secondary drivers

It may be less obvious that preventing infection is particularly important for children who are more vulnerable to infection. Such children include those with complex medical needs and may have reduced natural immunity or abilities to prevent infection. Children who are receiving medication that suppresses their immunity, such as those receiving chemotherapy for cancer treatment, or medication to prevent rejection of a transplanted organ are children who are more vulnerable to infection and require as much protection as possible. Children with chronic health conditions, such as asthma or diabetes can be negatively affected by viral illnesses.

Turning to the staff, reducing the spread of infection can lead to lower levels of illness, which in turn can promote better wellbeing, and reduce the levels of staff absenteeism. The drivers for preventing infections are illustrated in Figure 6.1.

In addition to the above reasons why preventing infection is important, another driver is how this can make a contribution in the reduction of the use of antibiotics.

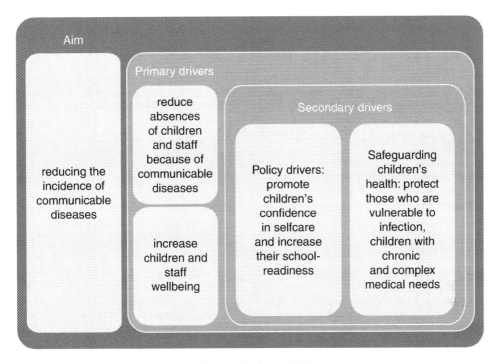

Figure 6.1 Drivers for preventing infections in early childhood settings.

Antibiotic resistance

When antibiotics were first introduced, which was in the 1940s, many of the serious infectious diseases that caused unpleasant illnesses and were frequently fatal became curable. However, antibiotics have been used inappropriately and this has caused the very concerning problem of some bacteria becoming resistant to antibiotics. It is estimated that 10m people will die by 2050 because of antibiotic resistance. Some of this problem has emerged because of doctors being pressured to prescribe antibiotics when they were not required. Another factor is the availability of antibiotics in some countries, lack of regulation in the dispensing and availability of antibiotics has meant they can be purchased without a doctor's prescription, which of course can mean that they are not necessarily the right treatment. Another reason that antibiotics are no longer reliable treatment for many types of bacterial infection is because the patents on antibiotics expired on many preparations, which means that they are available cheaply, this has the negative impact of pharmaceutical companies not reinvesting in research to develop the next generation of antibiotics.

Antibiotic stewardship

As knowledge about antibiotics resistance increases and their effectiveness is decreasing, it is imperative that we all share a responsibility to use the antibiotics we have available with great care. This approach is referred to as *antibiotic stewardship*; for more information about this, please look at the free, online course that is available, the link is at the end of the chapter.

Maintaining a healthy environment

Maintaining a healthy environment is a key part of preventing infection and requires careful thought to identify the ways and places where micro-organisms can multiply or be transferred. Developing policies that reflect the legislative requirements as well as the individual needs of a setting are important; this point will be revisited below.

Hand hygiene, as discussed above, effective hand hygiene, that is, hand washing and hand drying is an important personal habit to adopt. Good hand hygiene helps to remove micro-organisms that can be spread by touch onto surfaces in the environment.

Disposable gloves are to minimise the spread of infection and should be used when there is a risk of contact with bodily fluids, such as faeces, sputum and vomit. Disposable gloves should be used once, and only for one child and then disposed of, in addition, it is important to be conscious of what you are touching when wearing disposable gloves. Some disposable gloves contain latex which is an allergen for some people. Hand hygiene procedures need to be followed both before and after the use of disposable gloves. For further information, please see the Royal College of Nursing website for guidance, the link is below, about the use of disposable gloves.

Face masks became part of the strategy to prevent the spread of covid during the pandemic. There are mixed views about the use of face masks. The Lancet (Lifjering 2021) published an article stating that there is inadequate evidence to support claims that mandatory face masks contributed to a reduction in the spread of the virus. I would offer that the use of cloth masks, that do not fit correctly, are not washed regularly and are handled by the wearer, could potentially contribute to the spread of infection. The use of face masks by adults who work with young children, or with hearing impaired people is not advisable because they are a barrier to communication.

Toilets in education settings play an important part in relation to promoting good health. However, toilets in many schools are unhygienic and not well-maintained. Sarah Burton (2013) explored the literature relating to toilets in schools. She states:

> In some cases lack of cleanliness or poor toilet hygiene and usage represents a very specific risk of passing on infection and disease which can cause short term illness and absence from school. (p. 6)

Burton's review goes on to highlight how unhygienic toilets that smell, have blocked toilets, limited or no toilet paper, or with unreachable, dirty or no soap available, can deter children from going to the toilet. Children were reported as limiting their fluid intake in order to limit their need to pass urine, in turn can impact on children's health by causing them to be prone to developing urinary tract infections and wetting. In addition, inadequate fluid intake can contribute to constipation and soiling, all of these conditions can have long term consequences.

Food hygiene is important because food that is infected can be a source of infectious diseases. Therefore, training in the management of food hygiene is important for those responsible for the preparation of food.

Bodily fluids

Babies, young children and children with special educational and/or complex medical needs may have less control over bodily fluids such as urine, faeces, vomit, nasal secretions and blood. Therefore, having a procedure which ensures that there is safe disposal of such fluids is an important way of reducing the risk of infection spreading.

Routine immunisation

Immunisations are available to help develop immunity to many infectious diseases that are preventable infections, such as influenza, measles, meningitis, mumps, pertussis, pneumonia, polio, rubella, tetanus and tuberculosis. There are immunisations for children during adolescents to protect against other infections. Young people who are starting university are vulnerable to infections and need to be aware of the importance of ensuring that they are up to date with routine immunisations.

Terms used

Immunisation is defined as

> Immunization is the process whereby a person is made immune or resistant to an infectious disease, typically by the administration of a vaccine. Vaccines stimulate the body's own immune system to protect the person against subsequent infection or disease. (World Health Organisation 2019)

Vaccination is defined as

> A vaccine is a biological preparation that improves immunity to a particular disease. A vaccine typically contains an agent that resembles a disease-causing microorganism, and is often made from weakened or killed forms of the microbe, its toxins or one of its surface proteins. (World Health Organisation 2019)

Herd immunity

The World Health Organisation recommend a 95% target to achieve herd immunity, which is defined as:

> Having a vaccine also benefits your whole community through 'herd immunity'. If enough people are vaccinated, it's harder for the disease to spread to those people who cannot have vaccines. For example, people who are ill or have a weakened immune system. (NHS 2019)

Global initiatives

Globally, there are many initiatives to prevent infectious diseases spreading by promoting vaccinations programmes. Bill Gates (Davies 2019) describes how the Global Polio Eradication Initiative has helped to tackle polio:

> Take polio as an example. In 1988, there were 350,000 people in 125 countries being paralysed every year by polio. But that same year the world established the Global Polio Eradication Initiative to immunize children against the disease. Since then, we've seen a 99.99% reduction in cases, down to 33 cases of wild poliovirus last year. Today, the virus is endemic in just three nations – Nigeria, Afghanistan and Pakistan.

Providing vaccinations is an example of an impactful intervention which prevents the deaths of many children and improves the quality of their lives.

National initiatives

Many high-income countries have nationally organised childhood immunisation programmes. In some countries, it is a legal requirement for children to be immunised prior to starting school. In 2017, Italy made it a legal requirement for children to be immunised prior to starting school. In England, general practitioners are incentivised to meet set targets for immunisation. Despite the national efforts that are put in to achieving herd immunity in order to achieve eradication, there are continuing challenges to improving the uptake of immunisations by parents in order to protect children against preventable communicable diseases. This is referred to as 'vaccine reluctance'. This is a situation that is similar globally as there is a growing number of people who are being described as 'anti-vaxxers' because of their opposition to children being vaccinated against infectious diseases. The following sections summarise some of the high-profile cases that have emerged in the last 20 years or so.

Vaccine reluctance

Vaccine reluctance is a global threat to preventing the threat of infection. Vaccine hesitancy is attributable to what Tull (2019) describes as the '3Cs' (complacency, convenience, and confidence). Infectious diseases that were thought to have been eradicated and therefore are viewed as not posing a threat. Consequently, there can be a drop in the uptake of vaccinations, because of complacency. For example, the World Health Organization (WHO) has stated that England has lost its measles-free status.
   Vaccine reluctance is a global problem:

> one-in-ten children are not receiving any vaccines at all, there is more work to be done, and not just in the poorest countries. By 2030, nearly 70% of these children will be living in middle-income countries because despite relative wealth of these countries, their immunisation programmes are not reaching vulnerable populations and large pockets of inequities are allowed to persist. (Davies 2019)

Below is a personal reflection on how many parents lost confidence in vaccinations in England.

Personal reflection: the legacy of the measles, mumps and rubella case in England

Working as a practice nurse in the community in 1997, I was responsible for managing the childhood immunisation programme. This aspect of my work meant that I worked closely with Health Visitors to try and ensure that parents were educated in the reasons for immunisations. I started to work as a practice nurse when the aftermath of the Measles Mumps Rubella (MMR) scandal was still prevalent. A prestigious peer-reviewed medical journal had published the findings of research by Dr Andrew Wakefield where he claimed that the MMR was responsible for children developing autism and bowel problems. Understandably, the media coverage of this research caused many parents to stop having their babies immunised. This was a difficult period because the facts surrounding the case were not clear at the time and government reassurances were met with suspicion and fear. It Is worth mentioning that there were methodological flaws in the research design and Wakefield was subsequently struck off the medical register, meaning that he was unable to continue practising medicine.

Parental attitudes to immunisations

Public Health England commissioned a national survey of parental attitudes to the national childhood immunisation programme. The survey reported in 2018 that confidence is high for the majority of parents. However, there are several reasons why parents may not take their children for immunisations, which include:

* Cultural and religious reasons
* Hard-to reach parents
* Parents who work may have difficulty getting time to attend clinics
* Parental concerns about 'overloading' their child's immune system
* Concerns about the safety of immunisations
* Lack of knowledge.

Cultural and religious resistance to immunisations

Despite the evidence of the effectiveness of immunisations in reducing the number of cases of infectious diseases, there are groups of people who believe that they should not be given to their children. In England, the Human Papilloma Virus (HPV) immunisation programme was introduced in 2009 with the aim of protecting females from developing cancer of the womb. HPV can be passed on via semen. However, there has been reluctance amongst some communities because it is regarded as immoral to encourage young people to engage in sexual activity.

In July 2019, Public Health England reported concerns about the possible low uptake by some Muslims of a new influenza vaccination for their children because it has been reported to contain gelatine derived from pigs which of course is not halal.

Concerns about the suitability of vaccinations for some religious groups is a global issue, the following section examines an example from America.

Focus on America

The United States has a policy that makes it mandatory for children to have received immunisations before they start school. However, there has been a rise in the number of cases of measles in some parts of Brooklyn, a suburb of New York City. The extent of the number of cases has resulted in the mayor of the city declaring a public health emergency and has ordered all residents to be vaccinated. The outbreak started in the Orthodox Jewish community and has been 'fuelled by a small group of anti-vaxxers' (Kendall-Raynor 2019, p. 8).

Reaching parents

Some parents are regarded as being 'hard to reach', meaning that they are often unable or reluctant to access health services for their children, the following section examines an example of how the Australian government to parents who were not getting their children vaccinated.

Focus on Australia

Peleg (2018) presented the view from Australia regarding the uptake of immunisations by parents for their children. Despite this being a free service and despite there being reports of children dying as a consequence of preventable infection, it was found that half the number of children who were eligible to have immunisations, were receiving them. In order to reverse this trend, the Australian government's Department of Health introduced a 'No jab, no Pay' policy (2017). This policy meant that if parents did not take their children to be immunised, they would not receive any state benefits that they were receiving. Reasons cited for low uptake of immunisations included a lack of access to services. In a country that is as large and areas that are geographically difficult to access, this is a major challenge.

The tensions

What is the impact of media reporting on the uptake of vaccinations? According to Vanderslott (2018), the impact of anti-vaxxers is not as great on the uptake of vaccinations as the media reporting suggests. This can be partly explained by what is termed as the belief-behaviour gap', meaning that what people profess to believe does not always translate into actions that match the belief.

Different perspectives

As with all things, there are different perspectives to consider and Figure 6.2 illustrates the various stakeholders involved in immunisations.

1   View the case for and against immunisations from the perspective of the different stakeholders and consider their priorities.
2   Can you think of any other perspectives that are not included in the above diagram?

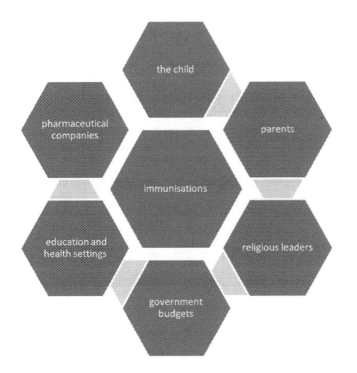

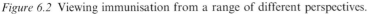

Figure 6.2 Viewing immunisation from a range of different perspectives.

Comment

The following section highlights some of the considerations in relation to the administration of immunisations. From the child's point of view, if children are not given immunisations, according to Peleg (2108) this contravenes their right to health. However, enforcing parents to immunise their children by withholding their benefit payments may be considered unethical. Therefore, there is a tension between parental rights versus the child's right to health.

Parental choice to not immunise their children can impact on other children, not just their own children. As stated above, promoting herd immunity will help to protect vulnerable children who cannot receive immunisations, for example, children who are receiving immune-suppressing drugs. Giving immunisations to immune-suppressed children is potentially dangerous, but if most children are immunised, this will reduce the chance of infectious diseases being spread. Thus, achieving herd immunity will help to confer the right to health on such children.

The motivations of religious leaders to dissuade parents from taking their children for immunisations appears to be founded in moral objections in some cases such as immunisations that are aimed at preventing sexually transmissible diseases. This is because in many religions, sexual relationships outside marriage and promiscuity are not acceptable. Therefore, this line of thinking may be understandable. A research study conducted in the Netherlands found that the orthodox Protestant religious leaders interviewed believed that giving immunisations 'interfered with divine providence' (Rijs et al. 2013). This is interpreted as meaning that giving immunisations is challenging the will of God.

From the point of view of a country's government, not having children immunised means that there is a higher risk of child mortality. And from an economic perspective, children who survive the effects of a communicable disease may be left with a legacy of disability which requires treatment. The impact of having the disease may continue into adulthood, thus meaning that employment opportunities are reduced.

Education and health settings who can reduce the incidence of communicable diseases are going to have higher attendance by staff and children. This has an economic benefit, as well as contributing to the wellbeing of individuals.

Pharmaceutical companies invest large amounts of money in to researching and developing safe vaccinations.

Summary

Professionals working with children in all contexts have a valuable role to play in preventing the spread of infection. It is evident that there are strongly held beliefs that can impact on individuals' understandings about the causes, prevention and treatment of infections. It is the responsibility of all professionals to be informed about how to work in sensitive ways with parents to encourage them to work together to prevent infections that impact on children's health and wellbeing.

The next section explores the causes and impact of parasitic conditions on children.

Parasitic conditions

Parasites live off a host and can infest the hair or skin of its host. Infestation is defined as 'the harbouring of worm or insect parasites in or on the skin' (Lawton 2017 p. 34). Globally, there are many parasites that cause infestations and diseases, some of which are less serious than others.

Insects

Malaria

Malaria is endemic in 109 countries and it is estimated that there were 219 million cases in 2010 (Williams et al. 2016). Malaria is caused by the plasmodium parasite and can be spread to humans by a single bite from an infected mosquito (NHS 2018). Malaria causes many deaths worldwide. Malaria can make people, especially children and pregnant women, more susceptible to other conditions, therefore preventing and treating malaria can reduce the possibility of other health conditions occurring.

The number of people affected by malaria is decreasing because of prevention and treatment measures, in particular, the work of the Bill and Melinda Gates Foundation has done a great deal to tackle malaria. Preventative measures require vigilance and economic resources. Anti-malaria bednets, those that have been treated with insecticides, insecticide-treated bednets (ITNs) are an important preventative measure, and UNICEF states that 40% of children in sub-Saharan African countries use bednets. However, in countries with limited resources, obtaining bednets is not always possible. Medication that prevents malaria is available, but again, it can be expensive to obtain, and the less expensive treatments can cause unpleasant side-effects. In addition, it is important to continue taking the medication in order to prevent malaria and compliance with taking regular medication can be difficult to maintain.

Malaria can be difficult to diagnose, especially as it can be dormant before causing symptoms. Therefore, if a child becomes unwell with a fever of more than 38 degrees, is shivery, has diarrhoea, vomiting, muscle pains or headaches and is known to have been travelling in an area where malaria is endemic, the possibility of malaria should be considered.

Lice can infest hair, both head and pubic, as well as skin. Itchiness is a common sign of infestation, not all who have an infestation of headlice will have itching, but some will experience extreme itching which can cause a secondary skin infection.

Scabies is derived from the Latin word 'scabere' meaning 'to scratch' and this is because the main symptom of the condition is intense itchiness.

Lice and scabies are not considered a serious health issue, although children's sleep can be affected because of itchiness. The intense scratching can result in a secondary infection, which is not to be under-estimated if a child also has eczema or is vulnerable to infections. However, there is a societal stigma associated with such infestations. Historically, they were associated with poverty, being dirty and associations with child neglect, but lice and scabies can affect all ages and social classes. But myths associated with how these infestations are acquired and who they affect are difficult to change, consequently, parents may feel guilty, or question their parenting, they may find it difficult to tell people around them, so the infestations may not be treated (Lawton 2017).

Worms

Worms are spread in dirty water and as Guest (2005) points out 'down a cup of dirty water in Nigeria, for instance and you may find yourself infested threadlike, meter long guinea worms' (p. 8). Worm infections in low-income countries are associated with other conditions such as undernutrition, poor growth and anaemia (Williams et al. 2016). In turn, these symptoms sap people of energy, leaving them unable to attend school and engage with education.

In countries where there is clean water available, good sanitation, the resources that help to minimise the spread of infestations and a temperate climate, such worms are not likely to be present. However, threadworms are a common parasite and 40% of children are estimated to be affected by threadworms. Threadworms are spread easily on toilet seat, under finger nails and scan be difficult to eradicate. Threadworms are problematic because they can cause intense anal and vulval itching which can cause sleep disturbance. Prolonged presence of threadworms can cause lack of appetite and weight loss. Treatment is available via an oral preparation, but good hygiene measures are also required to break the cycle.

The role of professionals in preventing infections and parasites

Preventing the spread of infection requires an all-professional approach (Richards 2017) and this includes professionals working in education. The following sections highlights some examples of how educators can play an important role in preventing the spread of infections and infestations in education settings.

Health education

Educators and other professionals working with children and young people are well placed to educate children and parents about the prevention of infection. This is illustrated by the findings from a Public Health England survey which was conducted to find out about parental attitudes to vaccination. An interesting point reported was that

> three times as many parents cited leaflets rather than online sources as their main source of information, suggesting that provision of high quality and accessible print materials remain vital to the programme's effective implementation. (2019 ND)

This point has important implications about the role of health and education professionals' role in displaying information relating to immunisations for parents.

Policies relating to the control of infection

Richards (2017) writing in the context of preventing infection in health settings, states that 'policies need to be owned and used by the practitioners who are accountable for enacting their provision, so regular update of the policy should involve a range of practitioners' (p. 36). This statement is relevant to practitioners working with all children and young people in all contexts. As well as involving practitioners, it is important to involve parents in understanding their role in preventing infection. The following sections includes an example of a policy in a day care setting for children aged 0–5 years. As you read the policy consider the following questions:

Questions

1   How does this policy help to prevent the spread of infection?
2   View the policy from the perspective of

- Practitioners
- Parents
- The child(ren).

Sickness and Ill health policy – Hollybush Nursery

As a nursery, we come across many kinds of illness. We have an obligation to children and members of staff to minimise illness and infection. Children should not be left at nursery if unwell. If a child is unwell then they will prefer to be at home with their parent/carer rather than at nursery with their peers. It is vital that we follow the advice given to us by our registering authority and exclude specific contagious conditions, e.g., sickness and diarrhoea, conjunctivitis and chicken pox to protect the children in the nursery. Illness of this nature is highly contagious and it is exceedingly unfair to expose other children to the risk of a condition. We stress that the following guidelines must be adhered to:

- *Collecting your child*
  If your child becomes ill at nursery you will be asked to collect your child. Although sometimes difficult, it is imperative that you collect your child as soon as possible

after being contacted. Hopefully, this will reduce the spread of infection within the nursery, resulting in healthier children and staff.

- *Prescribed Treatment*

  If your child receives antibiotics from your doctor, they need to remain at home until they are well enough to return to nursery. It is important that children are not subjected to the rigours of the nursery day, which requires socialising with other children and being part of a group setting when they have first become ill. If upon return to the nursery, the staff feels that your child is still unwell you will be contacted to collect your child (see medicine policy).

    Medicine will be administered at the discretion of the manager.

    Qualified staff will administer inhalers and steroids in accordance with doctor's instructions.

Common illnesses to be aware of

- **Eye disorders**

  Sticky eye/conjunctivitis etc. is highly infectious. If eye drops are given and there is **no discharge** *coming from the eye, children can return to nursery.*

- *Sickness and diarrhoea*

  If your child has either or both of the above, please keep your child away from nursery **48 hours** *after they have become symptom free. This can pose considerable risk at the nursery as these infections spread easily among children and staff.*

- *Hand, foot and mouth*

  Onset usually presents itself as a fever; symptoms usually consist of tiny blisters on palms of hands, soles of feet and cheeks, lesions in sides of mouth or on gums and occasionally blisters on buttocks. This is a viral illness and is highly contagious. Children will be allowed to return to nursery when they are well enough in themselves. This spreads easily among young children.

    Please note that this is different from foot and mouth disease which is found in animals.

- *Chicken Pox*

  Children are usually unwell before getting chicken pox. Small pimples usually appear over the trunk area first, after a few hours they will blister. Children can return to nursery when blisters are dry (usually 7–10 days).

- **Cold and flu symptoms**

  Children will often present with symptoms such as runny noses, coughs and high fevers. Children can come into nursery as long as they are well enough in themselves; however, if the child's symptoms get any worse then you will be asked to collect them. If your child has a high temperature the emergency calpol procedure will take effect. (see medicine Policy).

- **Head lice**

  We ask parents to regularly check their child's hair. If parents find their child has head lice we would be grateful if they could inform the nursery so that other parents can be alerted to check their child's hair. If staff notice your child has head lice during their day at nursery, you will be asked to collect your child and treat their hair. They can return to nursery once their hair has been treated. Please note that most treatments require 2 separate applications as well as combing to ensure that all head lice are removed.

We follow guidance given to us by Public Health England (Health protection in schools and other childcare facilities) and advice from our local health protection unit on exclusion times for specific illnesses to protect other children, staff and visitors in the nursery. Poster displayed in office.

The nursery has the right to refuse admission to a child who is unwell. This decision will be taken by the manager on duty and is non-negotiable.

If we have reason to believe that any child in our care is suffering from a notifiable disease identified as such in the Public Health (Infection Diseases) Regulations 1988. We will contact the Health Protection Agency for advice. We will also inform Ofsted of any action taken.

Reviewed/updated... ....

Manager/Deputy signature... ....

Comment

The aim of this policy is to prevent the spread of infections; in turn, this will protect adults and children from becoming unwell, or from experiencing the discomfort or side-effects of an infestation of a parasite. However, when the above policy is viewed from the perspectives of practitioners, parents and the children, there may be competing priorities.

From the practitioners' perspective, it is clear they have carefully thought about how to inform the parents of the children in the nursery about the commonly occurring infections that affect the children in the nursery. The content explains how the symptoms of the condition present in children and the actions that need to be taken in the event of these symptoms appearing. The policy is based on guidance from organisations such as Public Health England (2014) and National Institute for Clinical Excellence (NICE) (2009), thus demonstrating that the information is evidence-based and robust. The signatures and date at the end of the document indicate that it is a 'live' document that is reviewed and updated to reflect events that require a review and change of the policy.

From the point of view of parents, the information is clear and should help them to know what they need to do to prevent the spread of infection. However, in the real world, parents have other priorities and even though they may be conflicted about placing another priority, such as their work commitments. Consequently, a tension between the perspectives of practitioners and parents can develop, and the welfare of the child may become a lower priority. Such a tension is not easy to resolve and requires skilful handling. Having a policy that is carefully explained to parents may help to prevent situations where a child attends an education setting when they are potentially infectious.

From the point of view of the child, feeling unwell because of an infectious disease can impact upon their wellbeing and as is implied in the Hollybush policy, can affect their ability to be sociable and fully take part in their setting.

Summary

This chapter has explored the ways that communicable diseases can be prevented and highlights the responsibility that we all have to minimise spread. Improvements in our own practice and the way we model behaviour to teach children and young people good health behaviours have been highlighted. The tensions that surround immunisations have been illustrated and it is important to remember that the child's right to health may be diminished because of parental beliefs about immunisation. As professionals, we need to be sensitive to parental beliefs but at the same time be aware that the welfare of the children we work with is paramount. It is worth remembering that some of the practices that were advocated to reduce the spread of the coronavirus, such as regular and effective handwashing, are what we should always have been doing.

References

Australian Government Department of Health. (2017) No Jab No Pay new requirements fact sheet. Available from https://www.health.gov.au/resources/publications/no-jab-no-pay-new-requirements-fact-sheet, accessed 21 August 2019.

BBC News (2017) Italy makes 12 vaccines compulsory for children. Available from https://www.bbc.co.uk/news/world-europe-39983799.

Burton, S. (2013) Toilets unblocked: a literature review of school toilets. Available from https://www.cypcs.org.uk/ufiles/Toilets-Literature-Review.pdf, accessed 17 August 2019.

Cassell and Company (1895) *The Family Physician: A Manual of Domestic Medicine*. London: Cassell.

Davies, S. C. (2019) Annual report of the chief medical officer. Health – our global asset. Available from file:///C:/Users/jm39645/Work%20Folders/Documents/Child%20Health/Chief_Medical_Officer_annual_report_2019_-_partnering_for_progress_-_accessible.pdf, accessed 28 July 2019.

Guest, R. (2005) *The Shackled Continent: Africa's Past, Present And Future*. London: McMillan.

Kendall-Raynor, P. (2019) Measles outbreak: misinformation and poverty fuelling quadrupling of worldwide cases. *Nursing Children and Young People*. RCN Journals 31(3): 8–9.

Kolak, A. M., Frey, T. J., Brown, C. A., and Vernon-Feagans, L. (2013) Minor illness, temperament and toddler social functioning. *Early Education and Development* 24(8): 1232–1244.

Lawton, S. (2017) Skin Infestations. *Primary Health Care*. RCN Journals 27(10): 34–40.

Lijfering, W. M. (2021) Revisiting the evidence for physical distancing, face masks and eye protection. The Lancet. Available from https://www.thelancet.com/action/showPdf?pii=S0140-6736%2821%2901742-6, accessed 19 March 2022.

Musgrave, J. (2020) Preventing infection – not just now, but always! *Early Childhood Blog*. Available from March | 2020 | Early Childhood Blog (open.ac.uk). Accessed 19 February 2022.

Musgrave, J. and Payler, J. (2021) Proposing a model for promoting children's health in early childhood education and care settings. *Children and Society*. https://onlinelibrary.wiley.com/doi/full/10.1111/chso.12449.

National Archives (ND) The Great Plague 1665-66. Available from http://www.nationalarchives.gov.uk/education/resources/great-plague/, accessed 19 August 2019.

National Health Service (2018) Malaria. Crown Copyright. Available from https://www.nhs.uk/conditions/Malaria/, accessed 1 September 2019.

National Health Service (2019) Why vaccination is safe and important. Available from https://www.nhs.uk/conditions/vaccinations/why-vaccination-is-safe-and-important/, accessed 17 August 2019.

National Institute for Health and Care Excellence (2009) Diarrhoea and vomiting caused by gastroenteritis in under 5s: diagnosis and management. Available from https://www.nice.org.uk/guidance/cg84, accessed 29 February 2020.

Parashar, Nelson, and Kang (2015) Diagnosis, management, and prevention of rotavirus gastroenteritis in children. *British Medical Journal*. BMJ 347: f7204. doi:10.1136/bmj.f7204. Accessed 19 March 2022.

Peleg, N. (2018) Children's health between the private and the public: children's rights analysis of child immunisation in Australia. Presentation at Contemporary Childhood Conference: Children in Space, Place and Time. University of Strathclyde, 6–7 September 2018.

Priday, G. (2019) How to reduce the number of sepsis cases in the UK. *Nursing Children and Young People* 11(4):12.

Public Health (Infectious Diseases) Regulations (1988) Available from http://www.legislation.gov.uk/uksi/1988/1546/made, accessed 29 February 2020.

Public Health England (2014) Guidance on infection control in schools. Available from https://assets.publishing.service.gov.uk/government/uploads/system/uploads/attachment_data/file/658507/Guidance_on_infection_control_in_schools.pdf, accessed 29 July 2019.

Public Health England (2018) Parental Attitudes to vaccines survey. *HPR* 13(14). Available from https://www.gov.uk/government/publications/health-protection-report-volume-13-2019/hpr-volume-13-issue-14-news-26-and-29-april, accessed 17 August 2019.

Richards, S. (2017) Why infection control should be everybody's responsibility. *Primary Health care* 27(7):12.

Royal College of Nursing (2016) Hand hygiene. Available from https://rcni.com/hosted-content/rcn/first-steps/hand-hygiene, accessed 31 August 2019.

Ruijs, W., Hautvast, J., Kerrar, S., Van der Velden, K., and Hulscher, M. (2013) The role of religious leaders in promoting acceptance of vaccination within a minority group: a qualitative study. *BMC Public Health* 13. Available from https://www.ncbi.nlm.nih.gov/pmc/articles/PMC3668146/, accessed 1 September 2019.

Storr, J., Kilpatrick, C., Allegranzi, B., and Syed, S. (2016) Redefining infection prevention and control in the new era of quality universal health coverage. *Journal of Research in Nursing* 2(1): 39–52.

Tull, K. (2019) *Vaccine Hesitancy: Guidance and Interventions.* K4D Helpdesk Report 672. Brighton, UK: Institute of Development Studies. Available from https://assets.publishing.service.gov.uk/media/5db80f9fe5274a4a9fd6e519/672_Vaccine_Hesitancy.pdf, accessed 12 January 2020.

UNICEF (2014) Mosquito nets. Available from https://www.unicef.org/supply/index_39977.html, accessed 29 February 2020.

UNICEF (2019) Global handwashing day 2019: clean hands for all. Available from https://www.unwater.org/global-handwashing-day-2019-clean-hands-for-all/, accessed 18 January 2020.

Vanderslott, S. (2018) Anti-vaxxer effect on vaccination rates is exaggerated. The Conversation. Available from https://theconversation.com/anti-vaxxer-effect-on-vaccination-rates-is-exaggerated-92630, accessed 27 July 2019.

Vinck, P., Pham, N. P., Bindu, K., Bedford, J., and Niles, E. (2019) Institutional trust and misinformation in the response to the 2018-19 Ebola outbreak in North Kivu, DRCongo: a population based survey. *The Lancet Infectious Diseases*. Available from https://www.thelancet.com/journals/laninf/article/PIIS1473-3099(19)30063-5/fulltext, accessed 18 January 2020.

Williams, B., Goenka, A., Magnus, D., and Allen, S. 2016). Chapter 13 child and adolescent health. In Nicholson, B., McKimm, J. and Allen, A. (Eds.) *Global Health*. London: Sage.

World Health Organisation (2019) Smallpox. Available from https://www.who.int/csr/disease/smallpox/en/, accessed 18 January 2020.

World Health Organisations (2019) Health topics – vaccines. Available from https://www.who.int/topics/vaccines/en/, accessed 17 august 2019.

Other resources

The Open University (2018) Understanding antibiotic resistance. Online course. Available from https://www.open.edu/openlearn/science-maths-technology/available-now-understanding-antibiotic-resistance, accessed 17 August 2019.

The Sepsis Trust. Home – Sepsis Trust.

7   Children's mental health and wellbeing

Introduction

The quality of children's mental health is a global concern and children are increasingly being diagnosed with mental health conditions. In England, the Royal College of Paediatrics and Child Health (RCPH 2017) reports that 10% of children are being diagnosed with a mental health condition. The impact of the global pandemic is revealing that the restrictions and changes in routine have had a negative impact on babies, children and young people, particularly on their wellbeing and mental health. The increasing alarm and media reporting about children's poor mental health may give the impression that this is a new phenomenon, however, children experiencing mental health problems is not new. In order to contextualise the current situation, the chapter starts by exploring children's mental health from a historical perspective. The chapter will then explore the factors that influence the development of good as well as poor mental health. It also examines the complex issues that are currently impacting on children's emotional and social wellbeing and are causing concerns about children's poor mental health.

It is without question that addressing mental health in children and doing as much as possible to promote good wellbeing and in turn, good mental health is vital, this is important from the point of view of each individual and for society. In a report by the Chief Medical Officer in England in July 2019, it was stated that 'mental health is the orphan of the health care system' (p. 20) meaning that mental health is under-resourced, and of course for children who require treatments to support their mental health, it is imperative that they receive high-quality services. The current discourse about children's mental health tends to view the child as being vulnerable and society and the adults within society as being deficit. Whilst the context of children's lives undoubtedly contributes to their sense of wellbeing, the chapter highlights that there is much that can be done within society to improve children's sense of wellbeing and prevent poor mental health. As professionals working with children, it is part of our responsibility to challenge the discourse and examine some of the factors that are contributing to poor health. You are encouraged to identify what we can do to reduce the negative impact on children's wellbeing and in turn, improve their sense of wellbeing and improve mental health. It is also important to be conscious of ways to help to empower children to be able to promote their own mental health.

DOI: 10.4324/9781003255437-10

Terms used in this chapter

Medical terminology is like a different language and can be impenetrable and this can make understanding the complexities of mental health even more of a challenge. In order to attempt to demystify the language associated with children's mental health, here are some terms used and their definitions (Table 7.1).

Table 7.1 Terms relating to mental health

Mental health	We all have mental health, the issue is whether it can be described as 'poor' or 'good'.
Mental health issues:	Used to describe a variety of conditions children may experience, including mild, moderate to severe, and ensuing conditions ranging from anxiety or depression through to bipolar disorder, schizophrenia and eating disorders (Rosa and Smith CRAE 2018).
Psychiatry	The study and treatment of mental illness, emotional disturbance and abnormal behaviour.
Psychology	The study of the human mind and its functions.

The historical perspective

The current concerns about poor mental health in children would suggest that this is a new phenomenon; however, this is not the case. The realisation that children may be vulnerable to developing mental health conditions is one that has started to emerge over the last one hundred years or so. The history of children's mental health has developed as the sociology of childhood has developed; these two aspects are interwoven. This point is illustrated by the comment 'how soon can a child go mad? … obviously not before it has some mind to go wrong, and then only in proportion to the quantity and quality of mind which it has'. This comment was written in a psychiatry textbook which was published almost 130 years ago (Maudsley 1895). The comment conveyed the lack of understanding at that time about children's development and the belief that childhood was not a distinct life stage, and that children were merely adults in waiting. Another reason why it was thought that children could not be regarded as being mentally unwell is because behavioural problems were viewed as being caused by children being 'bad' rather than 'mad' (Rey et al. 2015). Children who did not conform to the expected norms of behaviour were often marginalised from society, sometimes becoming labelled in derogatory terms, such as the 'village idiot'. In the 1800s, lunatic asylums emerged and children who were regarded as psychiatrically unwell were institutionalised and removed from society.

In the late 1800s, there was a lack of clarity about the causes of mental health conditions in children. However, during this time, a growing understanding developed that children could be affected mentally by psychological damage caused by grief, such as melancholia, or to use a contemporary phrase, depression. Such psychological damage was recognised as contributing to behavioural changes in children resulting in mania or hyperactivity.

In contemporary times, the effects on children's mental health could be attributed to what we would now call adverse childhood experiences (ACE). During this period of intense medical discovery, epilepsy and other physical conditions that caused children's behaviour to be regarded as abnormal, became recognised as distinct from mental health issues. Prior to this discovery, children who had epileptic fits were viewed as being mentally infirm, or even possessed by evil spirits, a belief which continues today in some cultures. Partly because there were no treatments available to control epilepsy, such children were frequently institutionalised and isolated from society. Towards, the end of the 19th century, adolescence started to become recognised as a distinct stage of life. Puberty was recognised as a significant cause of insanity and Durand-Fardel (1855) in Rey et al (2015) highlighted the existence of suicide in children.

The first part of the 20th century was a time when new knowledge about children's development was created by many prominent people from several disciplines. Educationists, such as Susan Isaacs (1919) and the McMillan sisters (1930) were pioneers in foregrounding the importance of nursery education in contributing to human development. Jean Piaget, a psychologist and a contemporary of Isaacs, developed his influential theory of children's cognitive development (1936). John Bowlby who was a psychiatrist, started his pioneering work into children's emotional development shortly after the Second World War by studying the effect on children of being separated from their mothers. From this work, he developed his theory of attachment (1969). These peoples' work helped to shine a light on child development and helped to develop understanding of what could be regarded as normal and abnormal behaviour in children. However, it must be borne in mind that each child is unique and developmental norms should not be regarded as an exact expectation of what a child can or cannot do by a certain age. World War 2 (1939–1945) had a profound impact upon many children, their experiences included being evacuated to places of safety away from their families to live with people who were unknown to them. Many evacuee children experienced cruelty and abuse and consequent trauma. In Europe, children were displaced from their home country, and many were murdered, situations which are still experienced by children in places of conflict around the world.

The medical specialism of psychiatry started to emerge for adults in the 1800s, but child psychiatry developed as a specialism much later, in the 1950s in Europe. This was partly as a consequence of the work of pioneers such as the aforementioned Isaacs, Piaget and Bowlby who increased understanding of child development, as well as the findings from research that explored children's experiences of trauma. In response to children's experiences during the years of conflict, the United Nations introduced the Rights of the Child (UNICEF) which meant that children have become regarded as citizens with rights in many places in the world. Other significant events included the discoveries of therapies and medication which were safe to use in the treatment of children with mental health conditions.

Critical questions

1   How can looking at children's mental health through a historical lens help our understanding of the contemporary situation?

Comment

This brief overview of the history of children's mental health highlights that children have always experienced mental health problems. However, it is only in relatively recent times, that is, about 70 years ago, that mental health has become recognised as such, and that specialist services and treatments have been developed. The section summarises some of the key events that have influenced the shift in the belief that children are not capable of experiencing mental health problems to the contemporary situation in many countries, where it is recognised that children can experience profound mental health conditions. It is important to highlight that this view is not one that is widely held globally, some cultures and religions hold beliefs that mean they do not recognise mental health as an illness. Instead, the causes of abnormal behaviour are sometimes attributed to children being possessed by evil spirits (Prospera, 2014).

Defining mental health

In the previous section, you have been encouraged to examine children's mental health through the historical lens and you have been encouraged to appreciate the fast pace of change that has taken place in relation to children's mental health. Bear in mind that it is only about 70 years ago that child psychiatry became a specialism; however, we are now in the situation where children's mental health is of global concern and 10% of children are being diagnosed with a mental health condition. The restrictions caused by the pandemic have increased the number of children who experience mental health difficulties. As with many concepts, there are many definitions of what we mean by the term 'mental health' and below are some contemporary definitions:

- Mental health is defined as a state of well-being in which every individual realises his or her own potential, can cope with the normal stresses of life, can work productively and fruitfully, and is able to make a contribution to her or his community (World Health Organisation 2018).
- Child mental health, the complete wellbeing and optimal development of a child in the emotional, behavioural, social and cognitive domains (NHS 2019).
- A problem experienced by a person which affects their emotions, thoughts or behaviour, which is out of keeping with their cultural beliefs and personality and is producing a negative effect on their lives or the lives of their family (Patel and Hanlon 2017).
- An interpretation of illness and the medicalisation of behaviours considered to be beyond the norm (Burton et al. 2014, p. 4).

Critical questions

1   Do you see any similarities between the definitions?
2   Does one definition stand out as being more useful to you in your understanding of mental health?
3   How applicable are the definitions when considering children's mental health?

Comment

Definitions of mental health can be helpful in order to understand what the issues are. However, the definitions above suggest that mental health is viewed as being associated with abnormal behaviour, but this highlights the question of what can be viewed as normal behaviour? Understanding what behaviour is typical for a child's age and stage of development is helpful because behaviour changes as a child grows and develops; adolescents' behaviour can be affected by the influence of hormones. Undoubtedly, extremes of behaviour can impact on the individual's quality of life and especially in relation to children, can be problematic for parents and wider society. It is also important to consider that what is normal behaviour for an individual can be abnormal for another. This is partly because a range of factors such social, gender, cultural and religious influences can impact upon

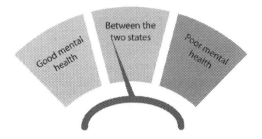

Figure 7.1 The windscreen wiper of mental health.

Source: Taken from Supporting Children's Mental Health and Wellbeing OpenLearn course, see link in the resources section).

views of what is normal behaviour. The definitions tend to convey a sense that the presence of poor mental health is static, and do not consider that abnormal behaviour that can be attributed to poor mental health can be a temporary situation. This highlights a difficulty associated with how long an abnormal behaviour may be exhibited before it is considered to be problematic and in need of an intervention. In relation to children, it is especially problematic to identify when a behaviour is an ongoing problem because of the rapidity of change in development. This highlights the importance of understanding each child's uniqueness and knowing each child, in order to identify when behaviour is problematic. Finally, the definitions tend to promote a utopian situation where all children will experience good wellbeing and in turn make a positive contribution to society.

It may be helpful to think of mental health as being like a windscreen wiper: on one side mental health can be good, but it can move across to the opposite side where it is bad. There is a great deal that we can do to keep our mental health on the good side of the spectrum.

Figure 7.1 represents mental health as a spectrum, with good mental health on one end and poor on the other. In a similar way to a windscreen wiper, mental health is not static, and it can move from one end of the spectrum to the other.

Creating the foundations of good mental health in children

There are a number of 'ingredients' which are regarded as important and necessary to children to support the development of good wellbeing and promote positive mental health. The following sections highlight these ingredients and explain their importance.

Meeting basic needs

Creating an environment for children which lends itself to them developing good wellbeing is a positive contribution to promoting good mental health. Human beings can be creatures of habit and children in particular gain a sense of stability by having a routine that meets their needs. The importance of providing routines that provide children with their basic needs are illustrated by Maslow's Hierarchy of Needs (1943). Adequate amounts of sleep is especially important for children's mental health. As well as the physical comfort of having food, fluids, sleep and warmth provided at regular intervals, fundamental to good wellbeing is the presence of positive relationships for children. Much of our understanding of the importance of warm relationships has been taught to us by John Bowlby's work on Attachment Theory (1969) (Figure 7.2).

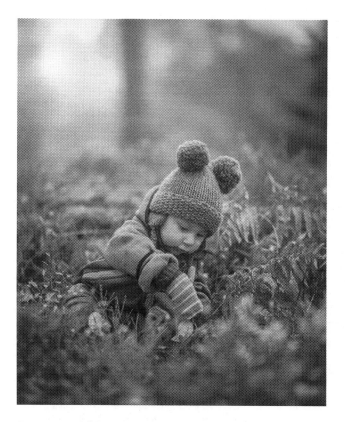

Figure 7.2 Child playing in autumn leaves.

Source: Unsplash IMG001716. Credit line: Janko Ferlic – Unsplash.

Promoting holistic development

While children's development is now viewed holistically, meaning that physical, cognitive, language, emotional and social areas overlap and inter-relate and influence each other, the aspects of children's development are that most directly influence wellbeing and in turn, their mental health are social and emotional development.

Social development, according to Doherty and Hughes (2009) is related to human's understanding of 'self', relationships with others and sociability.

Emotional development is related to concepts such as the ability to express and recognise emotion, the ability to develop attachments right from birth, as well as individual personality traits and temperament. Clearly, good physical, language and cognitive development also support the development of social and emotional development. For example, children who have physical mobility, the language skills and thinking processes are well-placed to develop good levels of emotional and social development. However, the context of children's lives is also vital to all areas of development, their environments need to enable their development and the relationships they develop need to be nurturing and positive.

Attachment can be described as an invisible emotional bond between two people. In relation to children, the attachment between mother and child is the bedrock of the child's development. John Bowlby is regarded as the pioneer of attachment theory; he laid the foundations of our understanding of the importance of emotional relationships for young children. Modern understanding of attachment theory has been influenced by neuroscience, Gerhardt (2004) in her book, *Why love matters* has foregrounded the importance of love and loving relationships for babies holistic development, right from birth. Such is the importance of the need for attachment, it has influenced education, care and health policy in England. For example, the key person approach is a requirement of the Early Years Foundation Stage (Department for Education, 2021) and is based on attachment theory, recognising that babies and young children need a special relationship with a caring adult in order to thrive. The Healthy Child Programme (Department of Health 2009), the universal approach to developing healthy children in England, highlights to Health Visitors how 'effective implementation of the Healthy Child Programme can lead to strong parent-child attachment and positive parenting can lead to better emotional and social wellbeing among children (p. 8).

Good wellbeing

If children's social and emotional development is good, it can be surmised that in turn, so will their level of wellbeing. Wellbeing is a concept that has many definitions, the Oxford English Dictionary define its meaning as 'the state of being comfortable, healthy or happy' (1998, p. 2096). There are many more, but there tends to be agreement that wellbeing refers to the quality of peoples' lives. Wellbeing can be viewed from the individual's point of view, or from the factors that influence the quality of our lives, such as our health, education, social or financial situation. There is growing awareness that whatever the outside view of an individual's life is, it is the individual's subjective assessment that is important in assessing wellbeing. Thus, suggesting that even if all ingredients that are necessary to develop good levels of social and emotional development are present, it is not always the case that individuals will have a good sense of wellbeing. Taking England as an example, many of the factors that contribute to good wellbeing are available to children as a given, for example, free school education, free health care and an infrastructure that is aimed at promoting children's wellbeing. Research conducted on children aged 8 and above by the Children's Society and the University of York (2017) has measured levels of wellbeing and the results indicate that many children's levels of wellbeing are not good. And this is having the effect of there being an increasing number of children who are presenting with mental health conditions.

Happiness is a term that is frequently associated with childhood; however, happiness is a transient concept, meaning that it is only ever temporary and therefore may be an unrealistic aspiration. Therefore, it may be better to improve wellbeing or strengthen resilience.

Resilience is the capacity to recover rapidly from difficulties. In relation to children, this can be likened to the ability to develop a cloak of protection around oneself, and not to take any slight or negative event personally. It can be regarded as the ability to move on emotionally from events that are unwelcome. A useful analogy to think about the meaning of resilience is that it can be compared to a ball's ability to 'bounce back', that is in response to an unwelcome event, one's emotions slump and can cause negative emotions such as despair, sadness and so on. However, the ability to correct one's emotions and return to a positive emotional feeling is helpful for good wellbeing. In relation to children and their ability to develop resilience, this would suggest that it is necessary for children to experience risk or adversity.

Social cohesion is cited as an important ingredient which makes an important contribution to humans' wellbeing. Social cohesion is linked to social development, meaning that the concept of being a socially cohesive group is based on the ability to develop and maintain positive relationships. Social cohesion can be described as the relationships that are present in a community, but each individual has a responsibility to act in a way that brings people together, the cohesion is like invisible glue that binds people together and in turn, this creates social cohesion. A utopian view of a socially cohesive community is one where children are able to grow and develop in an environment that supports their holistic development. This means having caring adults within and from outside the family who has children's best interests at heart. The environment within which the child lives enables their development, meaning that there are suitable indoor and outdoor areas for them to explore and enjoy, as well as high-quality health and education services available for children and families. Socially cohesive communities are safer societies, with adults aware of their responsibilities to keep children safe from harm. The society within which the child lives is structured in a way that is welcoming and nurturing for children and conveys to all members of the community that each adult and child belongs to that society.

In contrast, societies that are not socially cohesive, are often, but not always, in areas that are lacking in the features that contribute to a positive environment. Communities that lack leadership from adults who have a commitment to developing a good community spirit are often lacking in good services for children, such as playgroups and youth groups. Vandalism and crime contribute to fear and reduce individual's sense of feeling safe. Areas where crime rates are high frequently associated with drug dealing and excessive alcohol consumption. Such addictions can compound or provoke mental health problems and in turn this can impact on parents and their ability to parent their children, which can reduce the quality of relationships and increase the possibility of domestic violence. Living in poverty is a powerfully negative impact on children's health, and in particular, their mental health. The isolation of children who are living in homes where there is little money for the essentials in life such as food, where children feel unsafe and there is a poverty of love for the child can all lead to a sense of 'unbelonging' with negative consequences for their mental health.

Stress is a frequently used word and often in a negative context. However, stress is a physiological process, that is, it is the body's response to an event that requires action. Events that provoke emotions such as anxiety prompt the body to produce adrenaline, which is the fight or flight hormone. A hormone can be described as a chemical messenger, meaning that it relays a message to another part of the body. This origin of this response goes back to caveman times when humans had to be on high alert, to be aware of the presence of predators. In response to becoming aware of the presence of a sabre-toothed tiger who may snatch a baby for a snack, humans developed the mechanism to be able to respond to such a danger. The body released adrenaline which sent the message to various parts of the body to equip them to stay and fight or to run away. Whichever tactic was adopted, the body required help to respond, for example, adrenaline increases blood pressure so that oxygen could be circulated more efficiently around the body, which made running easier. If adrenaline was not released to act as a chemical messenger, then the body would not be able to respond and in caveman times, many humans would have been eaten by sabre-toothed tigers! Therefore, stress is protective and is necessary to keep us on our toes. However, ongoing stress caused by events that are unpleasant and unwelcome mean that the body is constantly producing adrenaline. This can mean that there is a constant feeling of anxiety and edginess. This can lead to a feeling of hyper-arousal, and in children, this can manifest itself in a variety of ways, for example, they may exhibit inappropriate behaviour. Children who live in homes where there is domestic violence are known to live in a state of hyper-arousal because of the anxiety that accompanies the threat of witnessing violence. Such ongoing states of hyper-arousal are known to lead to poor mental health as well as long-term damage to health into adulthood, such as heart disease, therefore, minimising excessive and prolonged stress is very important for good health in childhood and adulthood.

Self-regulation is related to the ability to cope with stress and manage their emotions. It is also associated with children learning to persevere with task that are difficult or challenging.

Factors that predispose children to developing Mental Health conditions

Children's level of wellbeing is dependent on many factors, most notably on the relationships they have that support them and the wellbeing of the child's family. Families are diverse and can be formed in many ways, some of which may appear unorthodox, what is important about the strength of the family is the quality of the relationships between the members of the family. Most important for children is that they feel loved and have a sense of belonging. According to research summarised by Newland (2014), the factors that contribute to good family wellbeing include parents with good mental health, have good social networks, a level of self-sufficiency and financial stability. Conversely, families' wellbeing is less good if they are living in poverty, parents have mental health problems, have chaotic routines and live in geographic areas which are inhospitable and have poor quality services, such as schooling. Therefore, the strength of the family is directly linked to the level of children's wellbeing and mental health. It is important to point out that many children live in families with less-than-ideal wellbeing and do not succumb to poor wellbeing and mental health issues. It is also important to be aware that many families who live in adverse conditions do not necessarily have poor wellbeing. When working with children and families, it is important to assess each child's context individually and identify the strengths that will inevitably be present.

Children who do not live with their biological parents and are in the care of the state, in England, known as 'looked-after children', are likely to have less than optimal health and this includes poorer mental health. The reasons for this are often associated with their experience of family breakup, removal from the family, the impact of the reasons why their birth parents were not deemed capable of caring for them may well have left deep psychological scars. It is likely that looked after children will have had a succession of adults caring for their welfare, rather than a small number of ever-present adults. Children who have fled from their country of birth to escape conflict and persecution and arrive to seek refuge in a foreign country, are likely to have experienced and witnessed trauma which understandably can predispose them to mental health problems. Such events are currently being described as Adverse Life Experiences, which is frequently shortened to 'ACEs'.

Adverse life experiences

The effect of adverse life experiences in early childhood has been well documented, such experiences include bereavement, abuse, neglect, family breakdown to name a few of the experiences that can 'cast a long shadow' (Rutter 1998) on a child's life which can continue into adulthood causing life-long psychological problems and increased risk of mental health problems. The restrictions and rules that were put in place to limit the spread of the pandemic will have been an adverse experience for some children. That is not to say that all children who experience adversity will be affected in this way, as outlined above, the presence of strong relationships and a supportive environment can do much to mitigate the impact of adversity on children. In Scotland and Wales, there is increasing attention being given to addressing the impact of ACEs on children, information relating to resources about this work is listed at the end of the chapter.

Adolescents and adverse life experiences

Much of the focus of this chapter has been on young children, this is partly because there is a great deal that can be done at this point to improve wellbeing and promote good mental health, the impact of which can have a positive impact across the lifespan. However, it is important to consider adolescents and their response to adverse experiences. Malone (2019) highlights that adolescents experience feelings of loss, grief and trauma differently to children or adults; however, the ways that adolescents express their feelings can mask the depth of feelings. This highlights how adults can underestimate the impact, therefore, it is important that professionals are aware that adolescents may appear unaffected, but the reality can be different. School nurses and teachers can play a vital role in supporting adolescents when they experience loss, grief and trauma.

Social media

The effects of social media on children's mental health are of concern, this is illustrated in research published in August 2019 by Viner et al. The findings which were published in the Lancet Children and Adolescents Health Journal were drawn from a longitudinal study and their conclusions are that children who frequently use social media are more likely to experience mental health problems, this is even more of so for girls than it is for boys. Social media carries a risk of being exposed to harmful content, in particular, cyber bullying. The research states that it is not just the social media that is the problem, but it is the accompanying lack of sleep that children and young people will experience because they are on social media late into the night. In addition, engaging with social media is likely to infringe on time that may be used for taking exercise, so they are being deprived of the positive effects on wellbeing that are associated with taking exercise.

This is a situation which is common to countries where children and young people can access social media and is of concern to governments around the World. In England, there is work in progress to produce an Internet Safety Strategy (HM Government 2018) which will set out more detailed measures to address harmful and illegal online content. This will include proposals on a social media code of practice and online advertising. However, managing children's access to social media cannot be solely a responsibility for government, there is urgent need for adults and especially parents and professionals who work with children to devise approaches to manage and limit children's access to social media. In addition, there is a great deal of work that can be done to educate very young children to learn about the impact of inappropriate use of social media.

Diagnosing mental health conditions

Diagnosing a mental illness in humans is not as straightforward as diagnosing a physical illness. For a physical illness or condition, as well as taking a medical history and carrying out a physical examination, there are a range of tests that can be carried out, such as blood tests, scans and X-rays. However, making a diagnosis of a mental illness is different because it is based on taking a medical history and can therefore be less objective. Mental illness is defined as behaviour 'outside the norm', however, deciding when a child is experiencing the symptoms of a mental illness and exhibiting 'abnormal' behaviour that can be attributed to a diagnosable condition is fraught with difficulties. One of the difficulties is that children's behaviour and response to experiences can be influenced by their age and their development. As children's development can be fast-paced and they can change very quickly, assessing whether children's responses are deemed to appropriate, or as Burton (2014) points out 'is considered to be beyond the norm' (p. 4) is a challenge. Another challenge to diagnosing or labelling a child with a mental health condition is linked to the above section where stress is discussed. As a society, we need to be aware that some of the educational and societal contexts within which children live their lives mean that they live in a state of hyper-arousal. For example, the concerns that children are exhibiting about testing in schools, the influence of social media and other health conditions, such as increasing levels of obesity are all factors that cause children to have increased levels of stress.

Childhood has changed greatly over the last couple of generations, for example, it is no longer the norm for children to play freely outdoors away from parental supervision as it used to be. The impact of the changing face of childhood means that children's access to open spaces is limited because of concerns about children's safety. In addition, the approach to a formal education in the primary stage, with less play opportunity and limited access to sport and outdoor play means that children may feel inhibited and possibly frustrated. We need to consider the role of adults in detoxifying the world we have shaped for our children.

Contemporary mental health affecting children

This section does not include a full description of each of the contemporary issues that are impacting on children's wellbeing, their mental health and in some cases causing children to have a mental illness diagnosed, detailed information can be found elsewhere, and some suggestions are made of where to look at the end of this chapter. What is included in the following sections are case studies that have been designed based on children with mental health symptoms and they illustrate some of the contemporary mental health problems that children can experience.

Case study: Macey

Macey is 14 and has been feeling increasingly lost over the last 2 or 3 months. Her parents had experienced a range of different events, the death of Macey's grandparents in quick succession; money problems caused by her dad's unexpected redundancy and just as she felt that life couldn't become much more difficult, her mum announced that she didn't love her dad any longer and a few days before Christmas, she moved out to go and live with someone she had met at work and with whom she had been having an affair. Macey was feeling really down, she is having difficulty in motivating herself to get up in the morning, partly because she is finding it difficult to sleep because she is sad and longing for her life to return to the way it was before her grandparents died and when she felt as if she belonged to a happy family. At school, she feels miserable, and this is partly because she doesn't want to tell her friends the reasons for her unhappiness, she is spending the long lunch break sitting in a toilet cubicle away from her friends. Her schoolwork is suffering because she can't concentrate and spends many minutes at a time staring out of the window.

Macey used to be outgoing and highly involved in all aspects of school life, her form tutor has noticed the dramatic change in her behaviour and is very concerned about her physical and mental wellbeing.

Questions

1   How much of Macey's situation can be attributed to a 'normal' reaction to her situation, some of which could be Adverse Childhood Experiences?
2   What can be done to support Macey?

Discussion

It was quite understandable that Macey will be feeling down and very fed up with the experiences she has had to endure. When do the normal responses to a horrible set of circumstances add up to become a mental health illness such as depression?

Symptoms lasting longer than two weeks or more merit a medical consultation with a general practitioner.

School could be a refuge for Macey, and there may be systems in place to support her, how education settings can support children with mental health problems is discussed in a section later in this chapter. For more guidance, the National Institute for Clinical Excellence issues guidance on many health conditions including depression in children and young people (NICE 2019) aged 5–19 years.

Refugee children and mental health

The movement of people around the globe because of war in their country of birth means that many children are in education settings who may not be familiar with the events that many refugee families experience. The following case study illustrates a refugee child's experience as he tries to become accustomed to living in England.

Case study: Shahram

The case study below is based on the experiences recounted by my former colleagues, Janet Harvell and Alison Prowle, following their visits to the French refugee camps in 2016.

Shahram is 8 years old and has recently arrived in England from Iraq. His family fled from Mosul following the death of their 20-year-old son, Omar, who was tortured and shot. The family paid people smugglers to help them leave Iraq, they wanted to join members of their family who had settled in London many years previously. They left Iraq with their immediate family members, leaving their friends, some family members, their family business and their home behind. They escaped with a small amount of cash, some jewellery and their mobile phones which contained the contact details of their friends, and most importantly photographs of happier times. The family reached Calais in February 2015 and lived in the refugee camp for 6 months because they were unable to complete their journey to England because of border control and immigration laws. The refugee camp was unsanitary, threatening, cold and bleak. Shahram's parents were anxious about letting the children go far from their tent because there were gangs of teenage boys who frequently fought with each other. So Shahram's life became an uneventful blurring of days with nothing to do; the most difficult aspect was coping with the boredom. Many hours were spent by the family queuing to receive small amounts of food or trying to keep warm and sleep.

Eventually, Shahram and his family were given permission to complete their journey to England. He was given a place at a primary school which was a 10-minute walk from his uncle's house. It was situated in a noisy street in London. The walk to school was at first exciting and being at school again after an 18-month gap felt like the start of a new life.

However, after the initial excitement of leaving the camp, reaching England and starting school, Shahram's euphoria ebbed away and he started to become anxious, tearful, withdrawn and socially isolated. The walk to school became something he dreaded, the shouts of the children and unexpected bumps from other children rushing along the pavement jarred his nerves. The people who looked like people from home worried him and he was confused about this because the familiar-looking people should have been reassuring. But were they people who would have been friends at home, or were they the enemy they had escaped from? The noise of cars backfiring reminded him of gunshot fire and when drivers suddenly accelerated and sped away, this reminded him of the enemies who shot his brother back in Iraq.

At school, the strange routines, unfamiliar food, unknown children, a foreign language all contributed to him feeling like a fish out of water and intensified his feelings of isolation. His teacher had 30 children in her class who spoke 7 different languages, there was a Teaching Assistant in the class. The TA gave him short periods of 1:1 time to try and help him to work out what the gaps were in his learning, hoping to help him catch up, but his poor English and her lack of ability to speak his language proved to be a barrier. Every social interaction at school became torture and the longed-for education in England intensified his feelings of failure and despair. Shahram found himself unable to sleep and eventually, his teacher realised that he needed help.

Questions

1   What are the key issues to address in order to improve Shahram's situation?
2   Who can help him?

Discussion

You may have decided that Shahram has clearly experienced many adverse experiences. Most notably observing the death of his brother, leaving his country of origin and having to endure long periods of boredom and lack of stimulation. The transition to an alien culture and feeling of social isolation all add to his poor wellbeing, you may have considered that Shahram is experiencing post-traumatic stress disorder (PTSD) because of the experiences he has had, his emotional responses to his new environment and his reactions to loud noises. PTSD is a common and understandable response to the adverse experiences that refugee children and families often go through. Clearly, Shahram requires professional help possibly medication to reduce his symptoms, and also therapy. Jabbar and Zaza (2017) report the benefits to refugee children who attended a rehabilitation programme which included drama and art therapy. This highlights the therapeutic benefits of creative activities and emphasises the importance of children having access to these opportunities in the curriculum.

Suicide

A concern relating to adolescents and their mental health is the risk of suicide, especially in relation to young males. In March 2019, the Samaritans (a charity that works to prevent suicide) reported that suicide, especially in young men, was associated with having had ACE. In particular, the numbers are higher in socio-economically disadvantaged boys, especially if they had experienced sexual abuse in childhood. Feelings of loneliness and not being accepted as part of a group is another factor that is a significant factor in decisions about attempting suicide. Suicide is a public health issue and with the right approaches, suicide is avoidable; however, it is important that adults and society are able to identify those at risk and even more importantly implement strategies and interventions that can avoid children and young people becoming suicidal.

Self harm is a term that covers a range of different acts that people do to deliberately cause pain or damage. The feeling that is experienced by people who self harm is sometimes described as a relief for overwhelming emotions. Please see guidance in the other resources section at the end of this chapter about how to approach a child who is self-harming.

The importance of education settings in promoting children's good mental health

The importance of babies and children having certain 'ingredients' in their lives to help them to develop a good sense of wellbeing and in turn how this can help to reduce the chance of developing poor mental health has been discussed. For many children, their home environment can provide these ingredients in the predictable routines at home where they experience warm relationships and interesting and stimulating play opportunities. However, many children live in chaotic homes where their parents find the struggles of daily life overwhelming, and this may mean that their children's wellbeing and needs are not given sufficient attention. For some families, this can be an on-going situation, for other families, they may go through periods of uncertainty and chaos because of bereavement, loss and other events that can impact on children's wellbeing. At such times, early care and education settings and schools can play a compensatory role for children, providing a secure and predictable environment.

For all children and young people, education settings, including pre-school, school, college and universities can all have an impact on all children and young peoples' mental health. The aims and principles of early childhood curricula lend themselves to supporting children's wellbeing. For young children, having the opportunity to engage with play can be therapeutic and the persistence that is required by children when engaging with some activities can help them to develop resilience. Outdoor play helps to stimulate the release of endorphins which are chemicals that promote a sense of wellbeing. Consequently, children who do not have the opportunity to take part in outdoor physical play may be predisposed to a reduced sense of wellbeing and consequently, poorer mental health.

Practitioners who provide high-quality education and care, working with children and families to support children's holistic development, have an important role to support and promote all areas of children's health, the benefits of doing so have long-term positive benefits in childhood as well as into adulthood. Working with children and their families to encourage children's independence and ability to self-care can mean that they will be more confident when they make the transition from pre-school to the school environment.

A whole school approach

The ethos of a school makes a significant contribution to children's mental health. A positive ethos is one which creates a welcoming environment which engenders a sense of belonging for each child. A whole school approach is where all staff are committed to every child's mental health and wellbeing as well as their educational progress. For more information about a whole school approach to children's mental health, please see Glazzard and Bostock's book (2018). Staff in schools are well-placed to spot the signs and to offer non-judgemental support, for more guidance about how to approach this sensitive subject, please look at the onlinefirstaid.com resources.

Managing change and transitions

Human beings are often fearful of change and for children who often have little control over some of the changes in their life, change can be especially worrying and cause anxiety. For this reason, there has been a great deal of research into how educators can best manage the transitions that children face. The transitions, that is, the physical movement from one environment to another can be as seemingly small as the handover of a baby from parent or carer to the key person in their setting. A 6-month-old baby who has not developed the concept of object permanence as described by Piaget (1936) and is experiencing separation anxiety will not know that his parent will return. The strategies that a practitioner can use to support babies as they separate from their main carers can have a profound impact on the baby's sense of wellbeing. As children become older and develop understanding and maturity, they may understand more about the transient nature of change, but change can be just as daunting.

Transition from primary to secondary school

Transition to secondary school is another significant milestone for children. In England, children can spend 7 years of their 11 years of life in the same school, so it is not surprising that the prospect of moving to secondary school can be daunting. Therefore, preparing children for the transition to primary school is important to minimise children's fear of the unknown. Children preparing to make the transition to secondary school often have concerns about bullying, friendships, harder work and stricter disciplines; however, research by Brown (2017) revealed that the move to a secondary school can be a positive experience for many children. She found that many children were making the transition from small schools with little space, many lived in cramped home environments, the generally larger secondary school environments and they flourished in the bigger environment.

These are encouraging findings which highlight that moving to secondary school can be a positive experience, and children are more likely to appreciate the benefits if they have a carefully managed transition.

Interventions to help children with mental health conditions

Interventions to promote good wellbeing and mental health are available in education settings. Children who have been referred to health professionals for their support are likely to initiate interventions. It will be important for health and education professionals to work together to understand the aims of such interventions and to ensure they are implemented in a consistent way.

As outlined above, education settings can offer opportunities to promote good mental health and wellbeing, and everyday routines in pre-school and school settings can be preventative. For example, giving children time to be heard and listened to are important for their sense of belonging and wellbeing and practices such as circle time or school council can be opportunities for children to express their thoughts. Of course, it is important for professionals to be available to listen at other times especially if children need to talk in confidence. For children who are experiencing symptoms associated with mental health, they may benefit from a range of interventions that can help to reduce the symptoms.

Hospital play therapists use art, building blocks and puppets to help communication and to allay the fears of children for many years, the principles of play as therapy has now crossed over into schools. The benefits of play using sand, art and Lego are being used for children who are anxious or find communication difficult.

Targeted nurture groups are another intervention that are being used in schools. Such groups are typically comprised of small groups of children who have been identified as those who are likely to benefit from having the input of an adult who has been trained to support children who are experiencing poor mental health.

Animal therapy is an approach that is often used to support children's mental health, dogs in particular can be supportive companions for children experiencing difficulties

Cognitive behaviour therapy (CBT) is a therapy originally used successfully with adults that is now increasingly being used with young children and adolescents but in modified ways to fit with individual children's developmental needs in terms of their cognitive, social and emotional skills.

Mindfulness is increasingly used with children as a relaxation technique and can include exercises such as yoga, breathing and yoga. It encourages children to enjoy being in the moment rather than becoming anxious about the past or worried about the future.

Medication – some children's symptoms may be so profound and have a significant impact on their ability to function to the extent that they require medication to suppress their symptoms. Prescribing medication will be a decision that is taken by a medical doctor.

Social prescribing is an alternative approach to medical prescribing and recognises that medication and other therapies are not necessarily the answer to some mental health problems. This is especially so for adolescents who have become socially excluded and are living in deprivation. Opportunities for young people to meet and socialise through community-based activities, such as sport, are being offered by Local Authorities and charities (Horner, 2018). Social prescribing is proving to be a successful way of using resources that are already available and highlights the importance of giving adolescents the right kind of opportunities to feel part of a community.

Reflection

- Consider the opportunities in education settings and within early childhood and school curricula that help to promote children's wellbeing and good mental health.

Comment

Reflecting on your responses to the previous activity, you may have identified that many early childhood settings and school environments have strategies and opportunities that can help children to develop good wellbeing. Routines that are predictable can make children feel secure. Engaging in interesting activities which are socially and intellectually stimulating can give children the opportunity to develop persistence with tasks.

The adults in education settings have a responsibility to children to be warm and consistent in their approach to children.

Summary

It is important to bear in mind that even if children live in supportive families, have strong relationships with adults and other children and have many of the foundations of good mental health in the context of their lives, they can still be at risk of developing mental health problems. On the other hand, children who experience ACE can develop remarkable levels of resilience and can be unaffected by their circumstances and experiences. There are key times and events in children's lives where the adults around them can do a great deal to support their wellbeing and make a contribution to preventing poor mental health.

References

Bowlby, J. (1969) *Attachment and Loss: Vol 1. Attachment*. New York: Basic Books.

Brown, J. (2017) The primary-secondary transition: the significance of space and place in their accounts of transition. Presentation at Contemporary Childhood Conference: Children in Space, Place and Time. University of Strathclyde, 6–7 September 2018.

Burton, M., Pavord, E., and Williams, B. (2014) *An Introduction to Child and Adolescent Mental Health*. London: Sage.

The Children's Society (2018) The good childhood report. Available at https://www.childrenssociety.org.uk/good-childhood-report, accessed 21 July 2019.

Davies, S. C. (2019) Annual report of the chief medical officer. Health – our global asset. Available from file:///C:/Users/jm39645/Work%20Folders/Documents/Child%20Health/Chief_Medical_Officer_annual_report_2019_-_partnering_for_progress_-_accessible.pdf, accessed 28 July 2019.

Department for Education (2017) Statutory framework for the Early Years Foundation Stage: setting the standards for learning, development and care for children from birth to five. Available from https://www.foundationyears.org.uk/files/2017/03/EYFS_STATUTORY_FRAMEWORK_2017.pdf, accessed 1 August 2019.

Department for Education (2021) Early Years Foundation Stage: statutory guidance. available from: https://assets.publishing.service.gov.uk/government/uploads/system/uploads/attachment_data/file/974907/EYFS_framework_-_March_2021.pdf, accessed 19 July 2022.

Department of Health (2009) The healthy child programme 0-5 years. Available from https://assets.publishing.service.gov.uk/government/uploads/system/uploads/attachment_data/file/167998/Health_Child_Programme.pdf, accessed 1 March 2020.

Doherty, J. and Hughes, M. (2009) *Child Development: Theory and Practice 0-11*. Harlow: Pearson.

Durand-Fardel, M. (1855) In Rey J. M., Assumpção Jr, F., Bernad, C. A., Çuhadaroğlu, F. C., Evans, B., Fung, D., Harper, B., Loidreau, L., Ono, Y., Pūras, D., Remschmidt, H., Robertson, B., Rusakoskaya, O. A., Schleime, K. (2015) History of Child and Adolescent Psychiatry. Available from https://iacapap.org/content/uploads/J.10-History-Child-Psychiatry-update-2018.pdf, accessed 15 April 2020.

Gerhardt, S. (2004) *Why Love Matters: How Affection Shapes a Baby's Brain*. Hove: Routledge.

Glazzard, J. and Mitchell, C. (2018) *Social Media and Mental Health in Schools*. St Albans: Critical Publishing.

Her Majesty's Government (2018) Government Response to the Internet Safety Strategy Green Paper. Available from https://assets.publishing.service.gov.uk/government/uploads/system/uploads/attachment_data/file/708873/Government_Response_to_the_Internet_Safety_Strategy_Green_Paper_-_Final.pdf, accessed 19 March 2022.

Horner, A. (2018) How social prescribing can help young people.

Isaacs, S. (1929) *The Nursery School*. London: Butler and Tanner.

Jabbar, S. and Zaza, H. (2017) Post-traumatic stress and depression (PSTD) and general anxiety among Iraqi refugee children: a case study from Jordan. *Early Child Development and Care* 198 (7): 1114–1134.

Malone, P. (2019) *Counselling Adolescents Through Loss, Grief and Trauma*. Oxford: Routledge.

Maslow, A. (1943) A Theory of Human Motivation. *Psychological Review* 50 (4): 370–396.

Maudsley, (1895) In Rey J. M., Assumpção Jr, F., Bernad, C. A., Çuhadaroğlu, F. C., Evans, B., Fung, D., Harper, B., Loidreau, L., Ono, Y., Pūras, D., Remschmidt, H., Robertson, B., Rusakoskaya, O. A., Schleime, K. (2015) History of Child and Adolescent Psychiatry. Available from https://iacapap.org/iacapap-textbook-of-child-and-adolescent-mental-health/.

McMillan, M. (1919) The nursery school. Forgotten Books. https://www.forgottenbooks.com/en/books/TheNurserySchool_10004448

NHS (2019) Child and adolescent mental health services (CAMHS). Available from https://www.nhs.uk/using-the-nhs/nhs-services/mental-health-services/child-and-adolescent-mental-health-services-camhs/, accessed 19 January 2020.

Newland, L. (2014) Supportive family contexts: promoting child wellbeing and resilience. *Early Child Development and Care*. doi:10.1080/03004430.2013.875543

National Institute for Clinical Excellence (NICE) (2019) Guidance for depression in children and Young People. Identification and management. Available from https://www.nice.org.uk/guidance/ng134, accessed 15 August 2019.

Patel, V. and Hanlon, C. (2017) *Where There Is Not Psychiatrist* (2nd Ed). London: The Royal College of Psychiatrists.

Piaget, J. (1936). *Origins of Intelligence in the Child*. London: Routledge & Kegan Paul.

Prospera, T. (2014) Witchcraft Branding and the Abuse of African Children in the UK: Causes, Effects and Professional Intervention. *Early Child Development and Care* 189(9–10): 1403–1414. 10.1080/03004430.2014.901015.

Rosa, G., and Smith, L. (2018). State of Children's Rights in England. Briefing 7: Health. Available from: http://www.crae.org.uk/media/126997/B7_CRAE_HEALTH_WEB.pdf. Accessed 6 May 2019.

Rey J. M., Assumpção Jr, F., Bernad, C. A., Çuhadaroğlu, F. C., Evans, B., Fung, D., Harper, B., Loidreau, L., Ono, Y., Pūras, D., Remschmidt, H., Robertson, B., Rusakoskaya, O. A., and Schleime, K. (2015) History of Child and Adolescent Psychiatry. Available from https://iacapap.org/iacapap-textbook-of-child-and-adolescent-mental-health/.

Royal College of Paediatrics and Child Health (2017) *State of Child Health Report.*

Rutter, M., Giller, H., and Hagell, A. (1998) *Anti Social Behaviour in Young People.* Cambridge: Cambridge University Press.

UNICEF History of Child Rights. Available from https://www.unicef.org/child-rights-convention/history-child-rights

Viner, R., Aswathikutty-Gireesh, A., Stiglic, N., Hudson, L., Goddings, A-L., and Ward, J. L. (2019). Roles of cyberbullying, sleep and physical activity in mediating the effects of social media use on mental health and wellbeing among young people. The Lancet Child and Adolescent Health. Published August 2019.

World Health Organization (2018) Mental health: strengthening our response. Available from https://www.who.int/news-room/fact-sheets/detail/mental-health-strengthening-our-response, accessed 29 February 2020.

Other resources

Department of Health and Social Care (2105) Future in mind: promoting, protecting and improving our children and young people's mental health and wellbeing. Available from https://assets.publishing.service.gov.uk/government/uploads/system/uploads/attachment_data/file/414024/Childrens_Mental_Health.pdf, accessed 1 August 2019.

Glazzard, J. and Bostock, R. (2018) *A Whole School Approach*. St. Alban's: Critical Publishing.

Jigsaw mental health resources for young people their parents and guardians. Available at https://jigsawonline.ie/?gclid=EAIaIQobChMI5fydp6-J5AIVFvhRCh2UQAbkEAAYAiAAEgKTKfD_BwE, accessed 17 August 2019.

Online First Aid.com (2021) How to help someone who you think is self-harming. Available from How to help someone who you think is self-harming (onlinefirstaid.com), accessed 7 February 2022.

Open University OpenLearn: Supporting Children's Menta Health and Wellbeing online free course. Available from https://www.open.edu/openlearn/mod/oucontent/view.php?id=106394&section=_unit3.1

8   Chronic health conditions

Introduction

This chapter explores the impact that a chronic, that is ongoing, condition can have on children and adolescents. The content explores some of the contemporary chronic conditions that affect children and identifies ways that professionals can work together to understand the impact and how education and care can be adapted to minimise such impact and maximise children's inclusion in their education and society.

What is a chronic health condition?

The term chronic can be defined as ongoing, in relation to health conditions, the term chronic means that the signs and symptoms are of longer duration than an acute condition, which is one of short duration, such as a common cold. For a condition to be chronic, it is normally one that lasts for more than 3 months and a condition that interferes with normal, everyday activities.

    Chronic conditions can occur in all of the systems of the body. For example, diabetes is a chronic condition that affects the metabolic system. The chronic conditions that are most prevalent in children in high and middle-income countries include physical conditions such as asthma, diabetes, eczema, epilepsy and sickle-cell anaemia. Mental health can be affected by a range of different conditions which include anxiety and depression (please see Chapter 7).

    Each chronic condition presents with a range of signs and symptoms. A sign is a characteristic that can be associated with a particular condition, for example, the classic signs of asthma include wheezing and coughing at night. A symptom can be best described as a feature of how the condition makes itself known that it is present in the child, again using the example of asthma, a child with asthma can experience shortness of breath.

Historical perspective of chronic health conditions

Until recent times, many of the chronic conditions that currently affect children were untreatable. In order to appreciate the complexity of chronic health conditions and the impact they used to have before modern treatments were developed, it is useful to examine the history of diabetes mellitus. This is a serious chronic condition which is affecting more children in contemporary times but can be managed effectively nowadays. Previously, children who developed diabetes mellitus would become dangerously ill and

DOI: 10.4324/9781003255437-11

they inevitably died. Diabetes mellitus, or Type 1 diabetes, is a metabolic condition because it is a condition that is caused by a deficiency of insulin which is a hormone (a chemical messenger) that is required to metabolise carbohydrates in food. Insulin is produced in the pancreas, a major organ of the body, however, some people are born with insufficient amounts of insulin. In normal function, when carbohydrates are eaten, the pancreas releases insulin into the blood stream in order to metabolise the carbohydrates which keeps the level of sugar in the blood within the normal, and safe, levels. Without insulin, the blood sugars in the blood stream cannot be regulated to remain within normal limits and they elevate causing high levels of sugar to circulate around the body, the elevated blood sugar level causes electrolyte imbalance which can eventually lead to cardiac arrest and death. In the 1920s, Banting, an English scientist, extracted insulin from Rosemary, a dog and successfully treated patients with her insulin, thus making a discovery that has saved the lives of millions of people who, without insulin, would otherwise have died. Following Banting's initial work, scientists learned how to retrieve insulin from pigs and cows so that they could be formulated into preparations that were safe for injections into humans. Further developments meant that insulin was formulated using human sources, rather than from animals, thus making it more acceptable for patients for whom the use of an animal product was abhorrent or unacceptable. It is still necessary to inject insulin into the body rather than being able to take an oral preparation because it has not proved possible to create an oral preparation because the enzymes in our stomachs destroy insulin, rendering it ineffective.

There is also Type 2 diabetes, when I trained as a nurse, diabetes mellitus was a condition that was referred to as being 'mild' for those patients whose pancreas produced some insulin, but not enough to keep their blood sugars within normal limits. Such patients could be managed by restricting the amount of carbohydrate in their diet, reducing their body weight and by taking tablets that stimulated the production of the insulin they were still producing. For many patients, one or a combination of these approaches worked. A typical patient with 'mild' diabetes was usually over the age of 40 and frequently overweight. However, as scientists researched the effects of Type 2 diabetes, it became apparent that the long-term effects of this type of diabetes had negative consequences on the body, such as an increased predisposition to developing heart disease. The profile of patients who develop Type 2 diabetes mellitus has changed since the start of the 21st century because there is a growing number of young children who are being diagnosed with Type 2 diabetes. This increase is associated with the higher levels of obesity in young children. This trend is extremely worrying because it means that the children who are developing this form of diabetes are being exposed at a much younger age to the risk of developing long-term complications as a consequence of having developed Type 2 diabetes.

Examples of chronic health conditions

The body's 'architecture' is made up of systems, a system being a connected part of the body. Another analogy is to think of each part of the body's system as a country's road network, each road and motorway play a part, and when all roads are open and traffic is running well. However, a failure of part of the system can have an impact on the rest of the system. Some chronic conditions can impact on more than one system, for example, cystic fibrosis affects the respiratory, digestive and metabolic system (Table 8.1).

Table 8.1 Examples of chronic health conditions

System of the body	Examples of chronic conditions
Cardiothoracic and circulatory	Heart conditions; sickle cell anaemia
Digestive	Coeliac disease; cystic fibrosis
Immune	Anaphylaxis
Metabolic	Diabetes type 1 and 2
Neurological	Epilepsy
Respiratory	Asthma; cystic fibrosis
Skeletal	Juvenile arthritis
Skin	Eczema
Renal	Chronic kidney failure; kidney transplant

Management of chronic health conditions

As mentioned above, a chronic condition is ongoing and this is because in many instances, the condition cannot be cured so that it goes away. Although it can be the case that a child may have a chronic condition for a long period of time and then the signs and symptoms can become less evident or disappear. Each of the contemporary chronic conditions that affect children has a range of different signs and symptoms that are typical of the condition. Therefore, having knowledge and understanding of such signs and symptoms is key to being able to recognise how conditions present in children. A guiding principle of managing the symptoms of a chronic condition is understanding how the impact of the symptom can be minimised so that the impact is lessened. For example, using the example of a skin condition such as eczema, having knowledge of what substances 'trigger' (or provoke) the symptoms of eczema means that such triggers can be removed, substituted or avoided. For children with eczema, soap can be a trigger which can cause itching, scratching, pain and possibly infection. The cycle of itching and scratching can have secondary effects on sleep, concentration and on the child's quality of life.

In order to manage chronic conditions and reduce the impact on the child, it may be necessary for the child to use medications which can minimise or suppress the symptoms. Medication can be given oral medicines, inhalers, injections, creams or rectal preparations.

Chronic health conditions in children

Each child is unique and similarly, the way that a chronic health condition affects a child can be unique to that child. Therefore, it is important to know each child and learn how to manage the condition in each child. The aims of management of a chronic health condition in children include:

- Gaining knowledge and understanding about the condition and the child
- Minimising the impact of symptoms that can affect many aspects of daily living
- Taking a holistic approach and considering the emotional effect on the child
- Developing and implementing policies in the setting: management of medication and procedures

- Maximising inclusion in education
- creating an environment that enables participation
- Working with the parents
- Working with other professionals

Personal reflection

After qualifying, I worked with children who had received kidney transplants, thus removing the need for nightly dialysis which involved using machines to replace the work of the damaged kidneys. The relative freedom that the transplanted kidney gave the children did a great deal to improve their quality of life. However, they still had to endure the restrictions of daily medication, hospital check-ups and the need to be cautious about contact with infections. The medication that suppressed their immunity to prevent their bodies rejecting the transplanted kidney, often had side-effects such as marked facial hair and swelling of the face. As children entered adolescence, it appeared that the impact of being different became more obvious and consequently, they often had very understandable reasons to rebel. The teenage years were often difficult years for them, they had another layer of complexity to add to the angst of being a teenager. Rebellious behaviour often manifested itself in missing appointments, stopping medication and angry outbursts. Another difficulty for teenagers was that as they reached 16 years of age, there was an expectation that they would transfer to adult medical services. However, in those days, there was little understanding of the need for a supported transition period. Consequently, it was usual for teenagers to have an appointment in the children's department one week and the following one in the adults' department.

Working with children who were experiencing health problems gave me insight into the impact on their families of having a child with an ongoing medical condition. Parents often had a range of difficulties to face; disturbed nights because of needing to attend to dialysis machines that were mal-functioning; missed days at work, or the inability to be in employment which led to reduced income and a loss of freedom and spontaneity because of the restrictions placed upon them by their child's condition. I saw many families come to breaking point because of the pressures caused by the added layer of complexity as a result of their child's health condition. I became aware that one of the pressures that some parents faced was because they were experts in their child's care and consequently had to be the source of information and knowledge about the management of the condition. In particular, parents of children with complex medical needs frequently became exhausted at having to repeat information to a range of different professionals.

The potential impact of living with a chronic health condition on children's development

Living with an ongoing health condition which requires constant attention to minimise its impact on daily routines has the potential to impact on children's all-round development. The following sections highlight some of the ways that their areas of development can be affected; however, it is important to point out that each area of development is inter-related and cannot be looked at in isolation.

Physical development

Whether, how, or if, a chronic condition impacts upon physical development depends to some extent on the condition. However, it is likely that all chronic conditions have the potential to negatively impact on physical development, although the degree to which this can occur can be more, or less apparent depending on the condition, the severity of the condition and how well or straightforward it is to manage the symptoms of the condition. Children with cystic fibrosis may have experienced failure to thrive which impacts on growth and this can result in physical development that is less than expected for a child of the same age. Other conditions can impact negatively in less obvious ways, for example, eczema is a common condition that is estimated to affect up to 11% of children and is the most common chronic skin condition in children. The word eczema comes from the Greek word meaning 'to boil' which illustrates the level of pain and discomfort that the inflammation accompanying this condition causes. The inflammation can be triggered by the skin being in contact with a range of everyday substances such as soap, sand, food and animal hair. Thinking about very young children, many of the learning activities that are designed to promote development include messy play, which involve sand, mud, water, modelling clay, which are all substances that are likely to trigger the inflammation associated with eczema. Consequently, children with eczema on their hands may be reluctant to engage with the activities that can help to develop fine motor skills, which may impair on physical development.

Emotional and psychological impact of chronic health conditions

Chronic health conditions can have an emotional and psychological impact on children, indeed Miall et al state that 'emotional, behavioural and educational difficulties are two to three times more likely than in healthy children' (2018, p. 163). Why this is so can be for a range of different reasons which will be explored further. Besides the physical discomfort that can cause pain and discomfort, some chronic health conditions, especially if they are not managed effectively, can potentially be life-threatening. However, even with careful management, 'breakthrough' symptoms can occur which in some cases can be life-threatening. There are several chronic conditions where this is the case, for example, as already discussed above, very high or very low blood sugars can be potentially life-threatening. Asthma can be unpredictable and asthma attacks are potentially life-threatening, indeed, in 2018, the Office for National Statistics reported that asthma was the cause of death for 22 children aged 0-19 (Office for National Statistics, 2021). Highlighting that chronic health conditions can be life-threatening is not meant to be alarmist, but it is pointed out in order to explain a reason why children may experience emotional and psychological responses to having a chronic condition. Children who experience the physical symptoms of a condition like asthma will experience the emotion of fear and anxiety.

Emotional and psychological responses to having a chronic health condition can arise from more mundane events, such as feeling excluded from activities because of the impact that taking part may have on the child. For instance, as mentioned above, a child with eczema may not be able to engage with some messy play activities because contact with substances such as sand, water or modelling clay can provoke inflammation which leads to intense itchiness and an overwhelming need to scratch. Eczema can be an under-estimated condition, however, it can profoundly impact upon a child. In this example, as well as the physical response, a child who is excluded from activities may feel a sense of rejection and social isolation. Eczema can be unsightly, children can develop wheals, crusting, inflamed skin which may bleed, all of which can be repellent to other children, and even adults; consequently, children may be teased, bullied or rejected because of the physical appearance caused by having a chronic condition.

It is also true to say that children with chronic conditions can become more independent and mature for their age because they need to learn ways to cope and live with a chronic condition and take responsibility for aspects of their care. Depending on a child's age and ability, those who are diagnosed with insulin-dependent diabetes are encouraged to manage their condition themselves right from the time of diagnosis. Living with a chronic condition often means that children develop deep pockets of resilience.

Medication and interventions to manage chronic health conditions

Most chronic conditions require interventions such as medication, which may be administered orally, via a feeding tube, by injection through the skin or even via the rectum. When the child is young, the administration of such medications will be the responsibility of the family or carers. As the child matures, they may be able to start taking responsibility for taking their medication and for some aspects of management of their care. However, it is important that they are supervised to ensure they are taking or doing whatever aspect of care they are starting to take responsibility for doing. As children enter adolescence, they generally become more independent for aspects of their life, and this naturally includes managing their condition. However, at the same time as they are entering this period of greater independence, adolescents can rebel against many things, and this can include the restrictions imposed upon them by their chronic condition. This can mean that adolescents stop taking their medication which has been prescribed to minimise, or remove, the symptoms of their condition. This can mean that they start to have breakthrough symptoms which can cause, discomfort, pain, long-term damage and can even be potentially life-threatening.

Adolescence

As children enter adolescence, the need to be aware of the impact of living with a chronic condition becomes even more complex. Adolescence is a time of change for children as they start to make the physical and emotional transition from childhood to the teenage years and living with an added layer of difficulty that having a chronic health condition can add to their lives can be understandably unwelcome. Ollerenshaw (2014) points out that 'risk taking and experimentation is a normal developmental feature of adolescence and this can be much more difficult for young people with a chronic illness' (p. 22). Such risk taking may include discontinuing the use of vital medication, such as inhalers or insulin injections, or experimentation with alcohol, which can be hazardous for adolescents without an ongoing condition but can be even more concerning for an adolescent with a condition that requires careful management.

Adolescence is a time when peer friendships can be difficult for all people at this age, however, living with the effects of a chronic condition can mean that the concerns that arise as a consequence can be very different from the experience of those who do not have a chronic condition. It is not uncommon for absence from school because of periods of illness lead to feelings of isolation. Also, the need to be mindful of their condition may mean that their friends have a different relationship, one that is more of a carer role. The following quote is taken from Ollerenshaw's book to illustrate the experience of one adolescent with a chronic condition:

> I think it puts pressure on friendships. It's tough on the other person if you're the one who always needs looking after. I hate that I need help. (2014, p. 22)

The needs of adolescents require professionals to have specialist knowledge of how to support adolescents.

Caring for adolescents with health needs is covered in more detail in Chapter 10. However, the health needs of adolescents with an ongoing condition require sensitive management to try and minimise the impact that feeling different because of their condition. It is probably true to say that most people do not like to stand out in ways that make them appear different from their peers or unusual, however, for adolescents, this feeling can be especially profound. Therefore, it is particularly important to respect their privacy in relation to what they may want to tell you, as well as helping them to maintain privacy when they need to carry out medical procedures.

For health professionals, there are some steps that can be taken to avoid the unwanted attention that absences from school for medical appointments can attract, such as running clinics after school hours or in school holidays. An inclusive approach to all adolescents can reduce the possible stigma of feeling singled out for additional support can be reduced by offering appointments for counselling to all at hospital visits.

Transition from adolescent to adult care environments

As children approach the age of 18, they are legally regarded as adults and are often transferred to adult health care environments; such transitions require some thought and sensitivity to enable the young person to adjust to what is a very different approach to managing their health. A child who has had a chronic health condition for most of their life may have received their health care in the same institution and possibly from the same staff for many years. Understandably, changing from a familiar and child-centred environment can be challenging.

Supporting children with chronic health conditions in education settings

The chapter has so far given an overview of the impact of chronic health conditions on children and adolescents, the impact on families of having a child with such a condition will be examined in Chapter 10. Children and adolescents spend a great deal of their lives being educated in pre-school, school or college. Therefore, the content of the chapter now turns towards examining how the complexities of living with an ongoing health condition need to be considered in relation to education settings. This part of the chapter looks at the care and support they need to receive in order to flourish in their education settings and to minimise the impact that having a chronic condition can have on their emotional, social, cognitive and physical development.

This section starts off by looking at Ingrid Miller who carried out a small-scale research project when she was a student at the University of Wolverhampton as part of her undergraduate degree dissertation to explore how children with Type 1 Diabetes (T1D) are supported in primary education. Below is an extract from her dissertation which presents some of the findings from her research, as you read the extract, consider the ways the school supports the child.

Research focus: caring for children with Type 1 Diabetes in a school

Interviewing the trained staff member, brought to my attention the level of care, knowledge and understanding needed to effectively care and support a child with T1D. He noted the importance of supporting other staff members and following each care plan as they are all different, *'Supporting staff with advice … different to the individual'* *(Designated Staff Member)*.

During the interview with the mother of a child with T1D, she spoke about some of the less obvious aspects of what she had to start doing after he had been diagnosed in order to manage her son's condition. She had to start checking labels on food packaging and mentally calculating numbers to ensure her sons' meals were balanced. The mum explained that she felt *'confused and angry with herself'* because of the impact of T1D on her and her son, however, she felt that some of her fears were eased by staff at the school as illustrated by this comment, *'school are supportive when he is ill and needs time off. I am always put at ease by any member of staff with regards to any concerns I may have'*. Mom worries about his attendance some days and stated that *'academically he is bright'*. Although her son cannot self-medicate, he can check his own blood sugar levels and knows when to request treatment if it is low.

The school takes measures where possible, to limit the impact of diabetes on the child's education, *'sometimes special measures are put in place where physical activities are involved'* *(Teacher 3)*.

MacMillan et al. (2014) discovered insights of facilitators and barriers to Physical Education (PE) and discussed some key areas including limited facilities for diabetes preparation and management. However, from my research, this limitation is not seen as the setting has made available the use of the medical room and ensured that most staff are trained in this area with staff and pupil having basic knowledge of T1D and how it may affect children. His study raised concerns from parents of the PE teacher's lack of knowledge on their children's condition. As stated before, within my work placement, the PE teacher is aware of these children and given information on the procedures to follow, *'It is important for information regarding T1D to be passed onto me, so we are not putting children's health at risk during exercise'* *(PE Teacher)*. He was notified of children with T1D as soon as he started working at the school and told whether the child could do their own blood sugar test.

The children will know there is a change as they have monitors that they regularly check. (PE Teacher)

Summary of findings from research

This study investigated how children with diabetes is supported in primary education from a teacher and parent perspective. Key findings suggest that there are still concerns with teachers when providing care and support. Findings from the research echo that of past researchers such as Musgrave (2014), McMillan et al., and Charalampopulos et al. (2017), on the lack of knowledge of children living with T1D and how it affects their education. This is reflected throughout the research and further highlights gaps found in past data. More should be done within schools to support staff working with children and their families. Teachers should be trained not only on their knowledge and ability to administer insulin, but also how to offer emotional support. Results show that there are still fears amongst teachers and that they felt more confident with their knowledge than they were with giving emergency care. Although regular training is provided, most teachers felt reluctant to administer these injections.

A review of literature also highlighted parental concern because the school their children attended did not disclose medical information to the PE teachers which could potentially put their child health at risk. Marshall et al. (2013) and Charalampopulos et al. (2017) both highlighted the need for improved staff support in their research and brought to light the concern of parents. Within my placement, all staff, including the PE teacher is well informed of children with T1D and the procedures in place to support both children and families. Working in partnership with medical staff, the school provides training on diabetes including safely and effectively administering injections. Building on parent partnership as well as working with different professionals will provide a stronger support network for children, parents and teachers. Along with past research, this remains an area of concern for most staff as they have fears of not administering it correctly.

Recommendation

While recognising the limitations of my analysis, this small-scale study has raised an awareness of the fears and concerns amongst staff members within the setting I conducted my investigation. It highlighted areas of provision for other educational establishments with an insight into the training needed to better support families and children living with T1D.

Reflection

Having read the extract from Ingrid's research, make notes in response to the following questions:

1   What are the considerations that need to be borne in mind for young children and adolescents with T1D in their education setting?
2   In relation to children and adolescent with a chronic health condition, what is the key information that is important to find out to help plan the care and education?

Comment: planning the care for a child with chronic health

As a professional working with children and young people with chronic health conditions, there are many considerations to take into account in order to plan for the management of their health. Many children will have an Education Health and Care (EHC) Plan that will have been developed when the child started education. However, not all will have an EHC, and as already discussed, it is very likely that the presence of an ongoing condition will present a child with some signs and symptoms which will need to be managed in order to maximise the child's inclusion in their education. Table 8.2 presents a series of questions that may be useful to you when you are planning the care for a child with a chronic condition. The second column gives you a space to write down the challenges presented by the condition and the third column is for you to make a note of solutions.

Table 8.2 A framework for managing the care and education of children and adolescents with a chronic health condition(s)

Questions: who/how/what/when/why	Challenges	Solutions
Knowledge and understanding of the condition Common signs and symptoms How does the condition affect the child? What triggers the signs and symptoms? How can the triggers be avoided? How can symptoms be treated? How much responsibility can he/she take for the management of their condition? What is the possible impact on other areas of development? How can you work with parents? How can you work with other professionals? How can you adapt or manage the environment to avoid triggers? What are the training needs of practitioners? How can inclusion be maximised?		

A framework for managing the care and education of children and adolescents with a chronic health condition

The framework is applicable to a range of different ongoing conditions and is designed to supplement and add to the information in an Education Health and Care plan.

The following section is the content of a handout which was prepared by a School Nurse for teachers in a school and it gives an overview of the chronic health condition, Juvenile Idiopathic Arthritis (JIA), summarising some of the key information that is helpful to plan for education and care. As you read the information, use the questions in the framework to help you to assess the needs of a child with JIA.

Information about managing Juvenile Idiopathic Arthritis

What is Juvenile Idiopathic Arthritis?

Juvenile Idiopathic Arthritis (JIA) is one of the most common causes of disability in children. It affects 1 in 1,000 children which means that around 12,000 children in the UK have JIA. We are not sure exactly why some children get arthritis, but it occurs when the immune system attacks the lining of the joints causing pain and inflammation. The aim of treatment is to get the condition under control and for the child to return to normal activities. It is important to note that children can have 'flares' of arthritis even after being well for some time. A flare happens when symptoms get worse or reoccur after being successfully treated. They can occur after infections, stress or treatment changes but the cause may not be known. Some children may grow out of arthritis, but some will continue to have symptoms into adult life.

Symptoms

A young child with any type of JIA or in a flare will present with pain, swelling, stiffness and heat in the affected joint. They may limp or walk with an abnormal gait, have trouble chewing or struggle with fine motor tasks. Other symptoms can include fatigue, fever, rash and generally feeling unwell. Even when symptoms of arthritis are controlled, the child may continue to have problems with pain and stiffness because of limited mobility whilst unwell. These children may require input from a physiotherapist. Some children with arthritis are at risk of developing a serious eye condition called uveitis and must be screened regularly.

Treatment

Untreated arthritis can cause irreversible bone/joint damage. The aim of treatment is to prevent this and enable the child to return to normal activities and join in with friends as soon as possible.

The first line of treatment is steroid injection to the affected joints. Young children usually need to have these under a general anaesthetic which will require a day or two off school. If these do not achieve satisfactory results, they may need to start on systemic medicines in the form of a subcutaneous weekly injection or an infusion. Injections can be done at home by a community nurse or the family but the child will need to attend hospital for infusions. These medicines can cause side effects such as nausea, vomiting, injection site irritation and anxiety. These medicines also require regular blood monitoring tests.

School and nursery

Most children with JIA manage well in mainstream school but may need help. Their needs should be assessed on an individual basis with input from Special Education Needs Co-ordinator (SENCo). An occupational therapist may be able to provide information and guidance on individual considerations for each child.

Considerations for staff include

Anxiety

Parents of a young child diagnosed with JIA may experience anxiety relating to the new diagnosis and treatment. Children may also experience anxiety relating to hospital visits, blood tests or injections.

Pain

It can cause tiredness, irritability and loss of concentration. Staff may need to give ibuprofen and paracetamol as prescribed. Often ibuprofen is prescribed at twice the normal dose for children with arthritis. Other ways to manage pain include rest and heat packs.

Side effects of medication

The child may feel nauseous or vomit as a side effect of their medicines. It is possible that nursery/school may need to be involved in managing the impact of this on the child.

Mobility

The family may need help getting to and from school, moving around school and using equipment. They may need extra help with dressing/undressing, toileting, etc. Children should rest when they have active arthritis but encouraged to join in with physical activity when symptoms are under control. This can be guided by the family and health professionals.

Hand function

Using pens, paintbrushes or tools may be difficult if finger joints are affected. Children may need encouragement to return to these activities once symptoms are under control.

Stiffness

Worsened after sitting for long periods so the child may need to be allowed to move around if needed.

Missing school or nursery

Due to symptoms of JIA or for treatment and investigations.

Further information

This is a general and brief guide to managing a child with JIA in nursery/school. It is important to keep close contact with the family to ensure the individual needs of each child are understood and met. It can also be useful to speak to the team caring for the family if the family is happy for them to share information. The clinical nurse specialist will be able to answer your questions and provide support. An occupational therapist or physiotherapist may be able to offer advice for specific problems for each individual child.

Comment

The information in the handout gives a general overview of the relevant information relating to this condition. The content helps to enhance knowledge and the questions in the Framework above can be used to understand the unique ways that such a condition can impact on individual children. The range of professionals who may be involved in the care of a child with JIA highlights the importance of professionals from health, social care and education working together to support the education and care of such a child.

Visible and invisible chronic health conditions

So far, this chapter has considered a range of different chronic health conditions that can affect children. What may have struck you is the range of different conditions and the impact that the presence of symptoms can have on children. Some conditions are more visible than others, it may be evident that a child with JIA has a condition if their mobility is affected; however, it may be less obvious that a child has diabetes. Hopefully, the message has been conveyed throughout the chapter that many ongoing conditions, whether invisible or visible, can have serious implications for children's health and wellbeing and as previously mentioned, may even be life-threatening. However, some chronic conditions may not be regarded as having serious implications for children because they are not visible and are not regarded as serious. One example is the condition known as 'glue ear'. The next section is an extract from Capewell's (2014a) research into glue ear, as you read the extract, consider the implications for the education and care of a child with glue ear, and identify ways that as a professional, you could minimise the impact on their education and care.

Glue ear: the case for it being a chronic childhood condition

Glue ear occurs when the chamber in the middle ear becomes filled with a sticky, glue-like substance. It is a form of conductive hearing loss as the sound waves are less able to travel across the middle ear chamber towards the inner ear and the hearing mechanism. Glue Ear or Otitis Media is one of the most common childhood complaints but is often overlooked as having any developmental or educational implications for children. This is despite it happening at a time when children are learning to speak and interact socially with others. It is acknowledged that glue ear is the most frequent reason for hearing impairment in children in developed countries leading to permanent hearing loss for some children (Rosenfeld et al. 2016). For most children, it will clear up spontaneously. However, it meets Mokkink et al.'s (2008) criteria for a chronic disease when it occurs: in children aged 0–18 years; is diagnosed on the basis of medical knowledge based on professional standards; Is not deemed to be curable; and continues to occur over a three month period or longer, which could include recurrence (p. 1444). Unlike other chronic childhood conditions, such as asthma and diabetes, glue ear is seen as somewhat trivial with little active monitoring by health care professionals and not included in regular health screening

The symptoms of glue ear is like the experience of many people when they fly and before their ears clear everything is muffled. Other people have described it as like hearing sound when underwater. The most effective way of simulating it is to put your fingers in your ears and try to understand what someone is saying at a normal voice level. For some, but not all children, it is accompanied by ear infections. The National Deaf Children's Society website (www.ndcs.org.uk) provides a lot of information for parents. Recent research by Avnstorp et al. (2016) suggests that the impact of hearing loss associated with glue ear may have been previously underestimated in terms of their ability to develop the ability to locate sound and to understand the spoken word in noise. They suggest that a more active approach is taken to monitoring and treating hearing loss and reducing damage to the ear drum.

In my own work (Capewell, 2014a), mothers often felt that they were not listened to or supported by both healthcare and educational professionals whereas their children were often able to express their own concerns. These included not always understanding what was said to them in the noisy environment of the classroom or how they felt their social relationships were impacted by the intermittent hearing loss associated with chronic glue ear. Ear ache often accompanies glue ear which can lead to parents feeling helpless when their child is in pain and they do not seem to be able to do anything about it. This is further compounded when the child has difficulty sleeping and may also demonstrate behavioural issues, such as anger and frustration (Rosenfeld et al. 2016).

Winskel (2006) suggests that those children who have had the condition from an early age with repeated bouts of glue ear are likely to have poorer reading and language skills when compared to their peers of similar backgrounds. Her findings may differ from others (Paradise 2007) as she used specific language tests. It is likely that with the use of current phonic testing and made-up words used in the UK early years setting these differences may be more apparent and could well warrant further investigation to see if a loss of hearing in such children is impeding their language acquisition. From a review of the literature (Capewell 2014b) a range of issues connected to chronic glue ear can be seen in children along with the relationship with parents. For example, some children can be seen to be overly dependent on their mothers and not want to leave them. In part, this could be because they have not developed the social skills of interacting with other children. However, it could also be because these children have not developed either the ability to locate the direction from which a sound is coming or to be able to block out sounds to which they do not need to pay attention. In my PhD study (Capewell, 2014c), one child described it as being 'attacked by the sound' and his mother explained how he resolved such issues by sitting under a table to form a natural barrier between himself and the incoming sounds. Strategies which may be effective for an individual child may be interpreted as odd by other adults, particularly in education. So the level of concentration required by a child with ongoing glue ear may lead to him/her to withdraw from other children and prefer to play by themselves. This may include playing solitary games such as puzzles. Because balance is connected with the ear then some children have poor co-ordination and gross motor skills. Some mothers identified that they felt upset and questioned their parenting skills when their child's behaviour was seen as perhaps indicating him/her being on the autistic spectrum. Another mother found that having her child diagnosed as dyslexic meant that he would be able to get the support he needed.

Although for many children this condition is short term and resolves itself by the age of ten, it does mean that the accompanying hearing loss can lead to them developing language and social skills more slowly. They may be exposed to less complex sentence structures and be more likely to not understand the pragmatics of language, but rather take a more literal approach. Those children with the condition continuing on into teenage years or adulthood but suffer from permanent hearing loss. In some cases, this can lead to behavioural issues as the frustration of not fully understanding what is said to them, and perhaps misinterpreting the motives of their peers in social situations.

There is an urgent need for greater understanding of this condition by educational professionals, especially those in the early years environment where it is very prevalent. It would seem to be beneficial for it to be included in training and to include strategies which can be implemented to minimise its impact in children's development.

Comment

Glue ear is a condition that may not be regarded as having long-term and negative implications for children's health, development and education; however, Capewell has presented compelling findings from her research that illustrate that there is a need to take this condition seriously.

Summary

How a chronic health condition, or conditions, impacts upon a child is, on the one hand, a unique experience; on the other hand, there are some commonalities that can help to mitigate the negative impact on children. First and foremost, it is important to understand the uniqueness of the impact of the condition on the child. It is also important to have detailed knowledge about the condition. The content of this chapter has illustrated that managing chronic conditions is complex. It is also important to bear in mind that some conditions are visible, and others are invisible. As highlighted by Capewell's research, an invisible and chronic condition such as glue ear can have a profound impact on children and all ongoing conditions can be a cause for concern. The adults around the child, both family and professionals such as educators, can play a significant role in making the lives of children with chronic conditions better. The approach and steps that can be taken to achieve this will vary depending on the age of the child and the level of maturity.

References

Avnstorp, M., Homøe, P., Bjerregaard, P., and Jensen, R. (2016) Chronic suppurative otitis media, middle ear pathology and corresponding hearing loss in a cohort of Greenlandic children. *International Journal of Pediatric Otorhinolaryngology* 83: 148–153.

Capewell, C. (2014a) The lived experience of glue ear - voices of mothers and young people. In 12th International Congress of the European Society of Pediatric Otorhinolaryngology: proceedings of a conference, Dublin, 2014. Dublin: ESPO.

Capewell, C. (2014b) Hear today but may not tomorrow – the implications of Glue Ear – research findings. *The British Psychological Society, DECPDebate* 150: 27–31.

Capewell, C. (2014c) The lived experience of glue ear: voices of mothers and young people. Unpublished thesis. https://ethos.bl.uk/OrderDetails.do?did=1&uin=uk.bl.ethos.668603

Census (2021). Deaths from asthma, respiratory disease, chronic obstructive pulmonary disease and flu. England and Wales. https://www.ons.gov.uk/peoplepopulationandcommunity/birthsdeathsandmarriages/deaths/adhocs/11241deathsfromasthmarespiratorydiseasechronicobstructivepulmonarydiseaseandflu englandandwales20012018occurrences

Charalampopoulos, D., Hesketh, K. R., Amin, R., Paes, V. M., Viner, R. M., and Stephenson, T. (2017). Psycho-educational interventions for children and young people with Type 1 Diabetes in the UK: How effective are they? A systematic review and meta-analysis. *PLOS ONE*, 12, e017968510.1371/journal.pone.0179685.

MacMillan, F., Kirk, A., Mutrie, N., Moola, F., and Robertson, K. (2014) Supporting participation in physical education at school in youth with type 1 diabetes: Perceptions of teachers, youth with type 1 diabetes, parents and diabetes professionals. *European Physical Education Review*, 21(1): 3–30.

Marshall, M., Gidman, W., and Callery, P. (2013)Supporting the care of children with diabetes in school: a qualitative study of nurses in the UK. *Diabetic Medicine*, 30, 871–877 10.1111/dme.12154.

Miall, L., Rudolf, M., and Smith, D. (2016) *Paediatrics at a Glance*. Chichester: Wiley Blackwell.

Musgrave, J. (2014) How do practitioners create inclusive environments for children in day care settings for children under 5 with chronic health conditions? Unpublished thesis: University of Sheffield.

Ollerenshaw, J. (2014) *Teaching Teenagers with Chronic Illnesses: A Secondary Teacher's Guide*. Sandy: Advance Materials.

Paradise, J., Feldman, H., Campbell, T., Dollaghan, C., Rockette, H., Pitcairn, D., Smith, C., Colborn, D., Bernard, B., Kurs-Lasky, M., Janosky, J., Sabo, D., O'Connor, R., and Pelham, W. (2007) Tympanostomy tubes and development outcomes at 9 to 11 years of age. *New England Journal of Medicine*, 356(3): 248–261.

Rosenfeld, R., Shin, J., Schwartz, S., Coggins, R., Gagnon, L., Hackell, J., Hoelting, D., Hunter, L., Kummer, A., Payne, S., Poe, D., Veling, M., Vila, P., Walsh, S., and Corrigan, M. (2016) Clinical practice guideline: otitis media with effusion (update). *Otolaryngology – Head and Neck Surgery* 154(1S): S1–S41.

Winskel, H. (2006) The effects of an early history of otitis media on children's language and literacy skill development. *British Journal of Educational Psychology* 76: 727–744.

Useful websites

http://www.arthritisresearchuk.org/arthritis-information/conditions/juvenile-idiopathic-arthritis.aspx

http://www.nras.org.uk/what-is-jia-

National Deaf Children's Society website (www.ndcs.org.uk).

9   Nutrition and oral health

Introduction

This chapter explores two contemporary issues that have a profound impact on babies and children's health and wellbeing, first, the importance of nutrition is discussed. Nutrition is a complex issue, and some of the reasons why good nutrition may not be available to all children are looked at. Babies and young children rely on adults to provide them with the food and drink; however, there are many factors that that influence the provision of nutrition to children, and they will be examined. As well as food intake, it is important to consider fluid intake; therefore, the chapter addresses some issues relating to healthy drinking. The other focus of this chapter is poor oral health which is another contemporary issue that is causing a great deal of concern because of the short- and long-term problems that can emerge because of inadequate oral hygiene. The chapter commences with a brief historical overview of childhood nutrition and oral health.

Historical perspective

In times gone by, children frequently went hungry and were often very small for their age because of inadequate nutrition. However, it is interesting to note that more than a hundred years ago, Margaret McMillan, a pioneer of nursery education in the east end of London, wrote:

> it is a mistake to think that all 'poor' children are under weight and underfed. Some are too heavy. And a good many eat too much ... the remarkable thing about the unnurtured is that they eat the wrong kind of food, and at the wrong hours and intervals ... this is not the only cause of rickets, but it is one link in the chain.
>
> (McMillan 1919, p. 50)

The language of this time jars with contemporary terminology, where McMillan refers to the 'unnurtured' is her description of the poor people in the area where the nursery was located. The comment about children being too heavy highlights that then as now, it was possible for children to be obese and poorly nourished. The comment about the wrong kind of food reflected what was available and affordable, and 'eating too much' was probably an indication that some children would be unsure about where their next meal was going to be available, what we now refer to as food insecurity. McMillan refers to the incidence of rickets, a condition which affects bone development in

DOI: 10.4324/9781003255437-12

children, it is caused by a lack of calcium or vitamin D. Sunlight is a source of vitamin D, and interestingly, when McMillan was working in the East End of London about a hundred years ago, girls were more likely to have rickets because they were more likely to remain indoors to help with small children and housework; therefore, they had less exposure to sunlight.

It may be difficult for people in many parts of the world who lived during the 1939–1945 war and the years of austerity during the 1950s to have observed the relationship that humans have developed with food. During the war, food was scarce, and people were encouraged to grow as much produce that they could to supplement the demand for food. The effect of such shortages, especially a lack of sugar and fats, meant that many people had relatively healthy diets and obesity was less of a problem. During the 1960s onwards, food technology developed, and this led to a proliferation of processed foods, a major advantage of this was that they were quick to prepare. The move away from food that was labour intensive to prepare meant that there was more time available, this was especially important for the increasing trend of mothers who worked outside the home, this was especially the case in high income countries.

Contemporary perspective

The contemporary picture of babies and children's nutrition is a complex one. We are probably familiar with media images of babies and children from low-income countries crying because they are hungry. But it may be surprising to some people that children who live-in high-income countries can be hungry and poorly nourished, but this is the reality of the many countries like the 4 nations of the UK in the 21st century. And the impact on the global economy following the pandemic is predicted to be a cause of increasing levels of childhood poverty which will lead to compromises being made in the way that children's nutritional needs are met. Childhood obesity is a critical contemporary health issue, with one in five children who start school at the age of five deemed to be overweight or obese. It is estimated that almost half of adolescent girls are deficient in iron, which can lead to anaemia.

As well as what children are given to eat, it is important to consider what they are given to drink, the provision of fluids to children is often overlooked, but require careful consideration (Howells and Musgrave 2021). Other health conditions associated with diet and nutrition include anaemia and vitamin D deficiency.

Stages of nutrition in pregnancy and childhood

Good nutrition is a fundamental component of life; however, each stage of human life, starting at pre-conception, presents a range of different considerations and challenges. Figure 9.1 illustrates the different stages when nutritional needs change from pre-conception through to adolescence.

Pre-conceptual nutrition

Good nutrition even before pregnancy has a positive impact on children's health. Taking folic acid before pregnancy (as well as during pregnancy) Inadequate intake

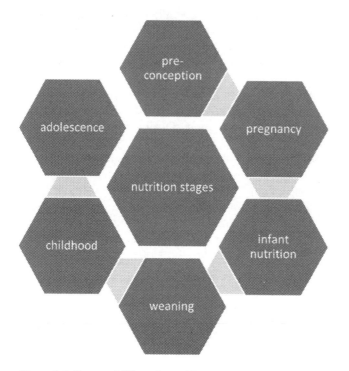

Figure 9.1 Stages of life and nutrition.

of folic acid is known to contribute to neuro developmental of babies, leading to spina bifida.

Antenatal health

Good nutrition during pregnancy is a key contribution to the health of children in the short and long term. However, many women's diet during pregnancy is deficient in the nutrients that are necessary for a health pregnancy and healthy baby (NHS 2020). Inadequate nutrition in pregnancy can impact on the oral health of babies and children.

Infant nutrition

The options for newborn babies are breastfeeding or bottle-feeding. Babies can be fed formula milk or breastmilk from bottles. Infant nutrition and the choices that parents make can be a controversial area.

Breastfeeding is widely promoted around the world as being the best form of nutrition for babies. Besides providing the right amounts of nutrition and hydration for babies, breastfeeding is reported to be effective in preventing obesity. According to the findings from Narzii and Simons' (2020) literature review of interventions to prevent or reduce obesity, breastfeeding is more effective than promoting healthy eating or physical activity interventions. However, breastfeeding is not many women's first choice of nutrition for their babies. In England, a quarter of all women never start breastfeeding, and whilst 75% do start breastfeeding at birth, by the time their baby is 6–8 weeks, this figure drops to 44% (Public Health England 2017).

There are several reasons that are cited as being barriers to breastfeeding, in the first instance, mothers report a lack of support to help mothers establish successful breastfeeding. Such support is especially important if babies are finding it difficult to 'latch on' to the nipple. Incorrect latching on can cause the mother pain, which can be caused by sore nipples or mastitis (inflammation of the breast tissue). As it's not possible to see how much a baby is taking from the breast, mothers can become concerned about whether their baby is consuming enough milk.

Mothers may not be aware of the full range of benefits that breastfeeding can give to their babies' health, therefore, educating and encouraging mothers to breastfeed their babies is an important health promotion focus. Support for mothers is important to establish successful breastfeeding, however, such support can be difficult to access. Mothers may find themselves isolated from family, friends and professionals, all of whom can play a part in supporting breastfeeding. The role of digital tools to support breastfeeding may help to provide the education and support new mothers to breastfeed (Bennett 2018).

Bottle feeding is usually for babies who are being fed with formula milk derived from cows' milk or soya. Preparing formula requires care, it is important to ensure that the correct ratio of water and formula is used, it's also critical that sterilising procedures for the equipment are followed to reduce the possibility of gastroenteritis, which can cause severe dehydration and death. It's easier to overfeed bottle fed babies and it can be tempting to push babies to take more than they really want or need.

Weaning (complementary feeding)

Weaning, or the preferred term, complementary feeding, is the introduction of foods, other than breast or formula milk to babies' diets, and is a significant milestone for babies. The introduction of complementary feeding is a time when healthy eating habits can be formed (Warren 2018). The World Health Organisation (2022) recommends that babies should be introduced to complementary feeding around 6 months of age. However, some countries around the world, such as some European countries, suggest that 4–6 months is the recommended age. Weaning has traditionally been parent led and comprised of spoon-feeding small amounts of pureed foods to the baby.

Baby self weaning is an approach to introducing complementary foods where the baby is given food similar food to all of the family, ensuring it is cut into small pieces, the baby controls what he eats as well as the amount of food that is eaten. Baby led weaning has gained popularity in some countries, such as the UK and New Zealand, possibly because these countries recommend introducing complementary feeding at 6 months, and this is the age that many babies are able to sit up and have the fine motor skills that are required to select and chew food. There has ben limited research into the effects of baby led weaning, but anecdotally, this approach could be advantageous to babies' development. Potentially, it can be a way of helping babies to have more agency over their food choices, as well as giving them an opportunity to develop their motor skills (Figure 9.2).

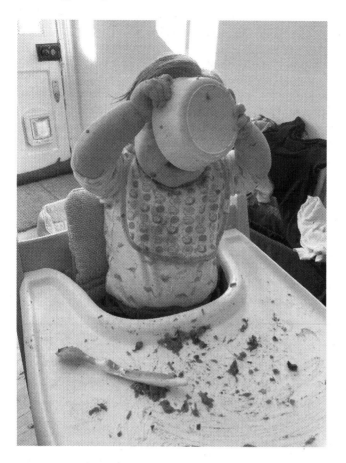

Figure 9.2 Jude: an example of baby led weaning.

Considerations for choices about the nutritional needs of babies

The previous sections have given a brief overview of the choices that mothers need to make about providing nourishment to their babies. There are some factors that can influence such choices, consider the following questions:

1   What may influence a mother's decision to breastfeed her baby?
2   What may influence a mother's decision to bottle feed her baby?
3   What are the factors that influence when and how a baby is weaned?

Comment

Although 'breast is best' is a widely held view, a campaign that was started by the World Health Organisation in the 1990s, there are many factors that can affect how successfully breastfeeding can be established. As outlined above, mothers can lack knowledge about breastfeeding, and may not have access to family, friends or professionals who are able to offer support and encouragement. The restrictions caused by covid meant that many mothers were socially isolated and professionals such as Health Visitors were taken away from their primary role which is to promote the health of babies and young children. The mother's health is a factor that can influence decisions about breastfeeding, some mothers may be receiving medication or treatment which can make breastfeeding difficult or inadvisable. Some mothers feel overwhelmed at the prospect of having sole responsibility for their baby's nutrition, they may feel that bottle feeding will mean that others can contribute and feed their baby. New parents may be embarrassed by breastfeeding, and they may find it distasteful. On the other hand, many mothers find that establishing breastfeeding successfully, is much more convenient. They may be able to avoid purchasing the equipment that is necessary to safely bottle feed, they can save the time that is needed to prepare feeds and to sterilise equipment.

The baby's health can also impact on whether successful breastfeeding can be established. A baby requiring medical attention shortly after birth can mean that a mother is unable to hold her baby and breastfeed. The mother may have a physical barrier that makes breastfeeding more challenging, for instance, a mother who has inverted nipples can mean that the baby has difficulty or is unable to latch on and draw down milk.

Practical considerations such as whether a mother is returning to work may deter some mothers from breastfeeding. Many mothers gain reassurance from giving bottle feeding formula milk to their baby because they know how much their baby is consuming.

Choices about how to approach the introduction of weaning, or complementary food, can be influenced by national policies. If parents are guided to introduce solid food at 4 months, parents are more likely to introduce pureed food that is fed to the baby, thus the baby has less independence and takes a less active role. On the other hand, if national guidance is to introduce solid food at 6 months, the baby is likely to have the motor skills necessary, for instance, the ability to sit up in a baby chair and be able to select what they eat from the food that is provided. However, the introduction of baby led weaning can be seen as having some drawbacks, some families may regard baby led weaning as time consuming and this may not fit with a busy schedule. This is because it may be seen as there is a need to prepare meals that are suitable for babies, which may feel like a restriction for some families. And as you can see from the picture of Jude (Figure 9.2), baby led weaning is a messy business which can produce additional washing and cleaning. Some parents can find introducing solid foods a time of anxiety, a common concern is that their baby may choke, and this can be a deterrent to the introduction of any foods that are not pureed.

For professionals, parents' choices about how they nourish their babies can conflict with medical and health guidance, thus creating a tension. It is important that parents are supported as much as possible, but of course, it is also important that their choices are not harmful to a baby.

Influences on healthy eating and nutrition

Ensuring that children eat healthily and gain adequate nutrition is a fundamental basic human need, and there are many factors that influence how this need is achieved. The following section explores some of the influencing factors from the perspective of the child, their family, as well as within society, both locally and globally.

The child

Parents can become anxious about their children's eating habits, and mealtimes can become a battleground. However, it is the case that some children find eating certain foods difficult. There may be medical or psychological reasons why this is the case. For example, children with autistic spectrum condition may be acutely sensitive to certain textures or colours which can result in them finding it difficult to eat certain foods. Children with cerebral palsy can have underdeveloped oral motor skills which can make it difficult for them to eat lumpy food (Ek and Hoglund 2016).

Children can be 'picky' eaters and show fear of trying new food, so called 'neo-phobia'. This can cause anxiety and difficulties for adults, both parents and profes-sionals who have responsibility for providing food to children. Tatlow-Golden (2019) points out that 'educators can bear in mind that children are not to blame for fussiness and neophobia' (p. 1). She goes on to explain that:

> fussiness and neophobia can be due to biological/developmental factors: (i) slower growth causing less eating; (ii) protective caution regarding new tastes at a time of first independent exploration; and (iii) increasing psychological autonomy. However, these behaviours can also be influenced by those around children, including their carers.

Tatlow-Golden's points remind us to think about the possibility of factors within the child which require consideration, however, she points to the responsibility of the adults in the child's life to be sensitive to the influence they can have on eating habits.

Family

Parents are frequently described as their children's first educators, and in the case of eating habits, the family powerfully influences how eating habits develop as well as on the quality of nutrition. The culture of the family impacts on how children are fed, not all families are able to have family routines with set mealtimes. It is beneficial to children to be encouraged to develop a healthy relationship with food. If a parent is concerned about their child's eating habits, mealtimes can become times of conflict and unhappiness, especially if the child is a 'picky' eater. It is important to remove the emotional dimension that can be attached to food, it should not be used as a bribe, a reward or for comfort. However, the reality is that food can be used for all these purposes.

Concepts of what constitutes healthy eating are influenced by factors such as living arrangements and housing; the absence of cooking equipment will restrict how meals can be prepared. Parents who are short of time may find that they have less time to prepare hot, nutritious meals that are eaten at a table with the family. Poverty con-tributes to poor nutrition, and food insecurity, that is, not knowing when food will be available affects 2.5 million children in the UK (UK Parliament 2021).

Community and global influences

The community that a child lives in can influence their food choices and in turn, their nutritional status. The powerful influence of advertising and its association with children's food is evident in many food products, and there are numerous products that are packaged in ways to appeal to children. Meizi et al. (2012) found in their study in Canada that communities with readily available take away food was found to have a negative impact on adolescents' eating habits. In many areas, there is a lack of local shops that sell fresh produce and food that is regarded as the basis of a healthy diet, and a lack of regular and affordable transport can make it difficult to go further afield to buy such products.

Multi-national fast-food chains that produce and market ultra-high processed foods play a significant role in influencing eating habits around the world. The United Nations Children's Fund (UNICEF) commissioned a study exploring digital food marketing in the Philippines (Tatlow-Golden and Boyland 2021), they reported:

> this food marketing monitoring study found that in the Philippines, social media is almost 100% saturated with marketing for unhealthy foods and non-alcoholic beverages. Advertising is appealing to 84% of adolescents. an almost entirely unhealthy 'advertised diet' is promoted to children and families, creating emotional associations of fun, love, sharing and health with these foods, and draws on the 'star' power of local sporting and media celebrities. (p. 5)

Conditions caused by poor nutrition

The following section gives some examples of some of the conditions that are affecting children's health that are caused by poor nutrition.

Childhood obesity

Childhood obesity is a global concern affecting 5.6% or 38.3 million children under the age of five. New Zealand has some of the highest rates in the world (Shakleton et al. 2018). As many as 10% of children in the UK are obese when they start school at the age of four (Narzisi and Simons 2020). In England, in 2015 to 2016, 19.8% of children aged 10 to 11 were obese and a further 14.3% were overweight (PHE 2015). In Southwark, a deprived area of London, 43% of 10–11 year olds are overweight or obese (Newton-Snow 2017). Obesity that starts in childhood has a negative impact on physical and mental health, and children who are obese are more likely to remain obese into adulthood.

Causes of childhood obesity

The causes of obesity are complex and identifying interventions to reverse obesity are challenging. Societal changes that have influenced childhood are thought to have contributed to the increase in obesity. Fears about children's safety has meant that children are kept under closer adult supervision, and this has reduced children's opportunities to play and take part in outdoor physical activity. Much of children's play and entertainment activities take place indoors and are likely to be more sedentary. The restrictions caused by the global pandemic meant that for many children their access to outdoor space was limited and their physical activity was curtailed. For children living in homes with no or limited outdoor space, and no access to outdoor areas in their education setting because of closures, this led to an increase in obesity. Many children live in an obesogenic environment, that is an environment that encourages weight gain rather than is conducive to weight loss; and to illustrate this, please read about Arlo.

Case study: Arlo

Arlo is 10 and he lives with his family in a high rise flat in a rundown council estate in London. His mum is a single parent and Arlo has four brothers, two older and two younger living in the flat. The flat is too small for a family of 5, there is limited space and the neighbours in the surrounding flats complain about the noise the family make.

The outside area is run down and unwelcoming, and the presence of young gangs makes the community feel unwelcoming and unsafe, so the boys do not play outdoors. As the school is very close to Arlo's home, he has a very short walk. At school, Arlo doesn't enjoy physical activity at break time, he prefers to sit and chat with some of his friends.

Arlo's mum is a cleaner at a local fast-food restaurant and must leave for work at 5 am; however, a bonus of the job is that she can take any leftover food home for the boys. This is an informal arrangement, and the owner pretends he doesn't know it's happening because he knows how vital this food source is to the family. She returns just in time to give the boys whatever she has brought home from work, often pizza or burgers before she takes the children to school. Arlo's mum is worried about leaving the boys because they aren't old enough to be left, but she feels she doesn't have a choice because she needs the extra money and the food leftovers. When the boys are at school, Arlo's mum works at a taxi firm answering calls.

To reduce the noise that the boys make, she encourages them to do activities that are sedentary such as playing electronic games or watching tv. Arlo's mum has limited time for shopping and cooking. The nearest cut price supermarket is a considerable distance and there is a limited bus service and even if she were able to find the time to go to the supermarket, she would find it difficult to carry the amount of food she needs to feed the family. Arlo's mum is severely overweight and gets out of breath if she carries heavy items. She has noticed that Arlo is becoming reluctant to leave the flat and when questioned, he says it's because he's worried about local gangs. Arlos's mum has also noticed that she is having to buy clothes that are made to fit a child aged 15 even though he is only 10.

Questions

1   What are the factors that are influencing Arlo's eating habits?
2   What are the solutions?

Comment

The reasons why Arlo and his family are either obese or at risk of obese are difficult to find solutions to reverse the trend. Arlo's mum's priority is to ensure that she can acquire sufficient food to feed her large family, and with limited income she relies on the free fast food. Without access to the food from her work, Arlo and his family may have to endure food insecurity. The family have limited opportunities to be physically active and have a sedentary lifestyle. The following sections examine some of the interventions that may help to prevent or reduce the incidence of childhood obesity.

Preventing and reducing the incidence of childhood obesity

With 10% of children labelled as obese when they start school at the age of 4 in England, there is a pressing need for actions to stem the progression of obesity. As Karzini and Simons (2020) assert, the first 5 years of a child's life is an important time to focus on preventing obesity. The need for interventions that start very early to prevent and reduce childhood obesity is a health imperative. However, identifying what works is difficult to assess because many studies do not have long term follow up to monitor the success in addressing the problem.

Finding solutions to the epidemic of obesity in childhood has occupied researchers around the world. In England, Narzisi and Simons (2021) concluded in their systematic literature to identify interventions that prevent or reduce obesity in children from birth to 5 years of age:

> A particularly influential time period appears to be new motherhood when mothers are receptive to health messages, as exemplified by the studies focusing on infant feeding and weaning practices. The ability to influence obesity risk factors at this early age suggests a need for universal provision of engaging infant nutrition practices, but particularly to families living in areas of deprivation. (p. 330)

As highlighted in the sections in this chapter about the choices available to mothers for their babies, establishing breastfeeding can be challenging and even impossible for some mothers. And similarly, the introduction of complementary foods, or weaning, is not always straightforward.

A community approach is needed to reduce childhood obesity (Office for Health Improvement and Disparities 2022) which includes the layers around children to include home, education setting and services.

Education settings are ideally placed to provide an environment that promotes healthy eating. Other strategies that are thought to reduce the factors that contribute to an obesogenic environment are to limit the advertising of less healthy food. In England, certain soft drinks are liable for a sugar tax which is aimed at reducing the consumption of high calorie and high sugar drinks (HM Treasury 2018).

The reasons why there are so many children who are obese and overweight are complex, so this makes finding solutions to reversing and preventing childhood obesity very difficult. While there is a need for adults to take responsibility for achieving this aim, it is critical that interventions are conducted in sensitive ways and without judgement.

Underweight children

While there is increased awareness and attention given to overweight and obese children, it is important to be aware that there are children who are underweight. Sometimes children's diets can contain too much wholegrain foods, or children's intake of carbonated drink can make them feel full and they may not feel hungry, and consequently they can miss out on the calories they need. An underweight child may be a sign of neglect. Children with eating disorders can be underweight.

Vitamin D insufficiency

Vitamin D is present in certain foods and by sunlight; it is required to absorb calcium from our diets and is essential for the healthy development and growth of the skeleton. Skeletal development happens mainly in infancy, childhood and adolescence, so large amounts are needed. Inadequate exposure to sunlight is another cause of Vitamin D insufficiency, this can be caused because of climate, or as a consequence of the use of sun block cream used to avoid the sun rays coming into direct contact with skin. Vitamin D insufficiency is a global problem, with many children, 'irrespective of diet, climate and skin tone' (Bentley 2015, p. 31) developing health problems. Rickets is one such problem, this is where bones fail to form properly and are weak, causing deformities that if not corrected before adolescence, can be irreversible.

Providing babies and children with oral Vitamin D supplements is an intervention that is recommended by the National Institute for Health and Care Excellence (2014) to ensure that babies and children receive adequate amounts of Vitamin D. Another consideration is to ensure that children are exposed to safe levels of sunlight, carefully balancing the time of exposure with the need to reduce the risk of skin damage that can lead to skin cancer.

Childhood anaemia is caused by insufficient intake of iron in the diet. Iron is needed by red blood cells to transport oxygen around the body, insufficient iron intake leads to reduced oxygen which can cause tiredness. Common causes of anaemia are delayed weaning or a diet that is low in iron containing foods such as red meat.

Dietary restriction

The provision of a healthy diet to babies and children can present many challenges, for some children, there are additional considerations related to them having their diets restricted for a range of reasons. One reason for dietary restriction is the presence of a medical condition such as an allergy or intolerance. Examples of other health conditions that require dietary restriction include diabetes, coeliac disease and cystic fibrosis. Another reason for dietary retraction is because of parental choice.

Allergy and dietary restriction

Allergic disease is a contemporary health issues that affects people in all areas of the world. In the UK, hospital admissions because of allergy to foods 'has increased fivefold between 1909–2007' (Gupta et al. 2007).

Allergy to substances can cause anaphylaxis, which is a severe reaction to foods and substances. Common foods that can cause a severe and potentially life-threatening reaction include nuts, sesame, strawberries, and kiwi. It is estimated that allergy to cow's milk affects between 2% and 7% of babies who are fed using formula milk.

Managing food allergy is an ongoing commitment and according to the Royal College of Paediatrics and Child Heath (2017) that can impair the quality of life of those affected.

When children are young, parents take the responsibility of managing dietary restrictions, although this responsibility is not taken in isolation because as children develop and understand more about the potential implications of eating a substance or food that they are allergic to, the management can become a shared responsibility. And research has revealed the critical role that early childhood educators can play in managing dietary restriction and avoiding the possibility of exposing children to allergenic foods (Musgrave 2014).

Adolescence can be a time where many young people want to fit in with their peers and are keen not to appear different. Trower and Gettings (2015) point out that for adolescents, eating food with their peers is a normal social activity Therefore, having a dietary restriction for at this time of life can add an unwelcome layer of complication. The need for careful dietary management would appear to be imperative and common sense would suggest that for long term health and wellbeing, dietary compliance is a good decision to take. But for young people, the need to be like their peers and to eat spontaneously or in a similar way to them can be far more important than considering the long-term complications. In relation to anaphylaxis, the likelihood of the perception is that risk-taking behaviour increases, and such behaviour can lead to a fatal anaphylactic reaction. Adolescents taking risks with food they are allergic to, is a problem as they are at higher risk of dying from anaphylaxis than younger children (Marrs and Lack 2013).

For those who are severely allergic to certain foods, the problem is that on occasions, food labelling is inadequate and hidden or undeclared ingredients have been a cause of fatal anaphylaxis. In England, a 15-year-old girl died after eating a baguette that contained sesame, a product that caused her to go into anaphylactic shock; however, sesame was an undeclared ingredient. Natalie Ednan-Laperouse's death was a consequence of unclear food labelling which led to a change in the laws about food labelling (Gov.Uk 2021).

Chronic health conditions and dietary restriction

There are many medical conditions that require dietary restriction to manage the symptoms and to reduce the chance of long-term damage. For example, for people with diabetes mellitus, controlling the intake of carbohydrate in the diet, and balancing the dose of insulin and the amount of physical activity is a key part of day-to-day management of this condition. The need for such control can take away opportunities that may arise to take part in spontaneous decisions to eat with friends. This balancing act between carbohydrate intake, insulin dose and level of physical activity requires a lifelong commitment to keep blood sugar levels within a range that is regarded as normal. Abnormal levels of sugar in the blood, especially spikes that rise above and then go below the normal can lead to complications of the major organs of the body. Blood vessel damage can lead to kidney failure, meaning that dialysis, or a kidney transplant is required to keep the person alive.

Coeliac disease is a chronic autoimmune disease which is managed by the removal of gluten from the child's diet. Gluten is found in wheat, barley and rye, meaning that many staple foods such as bread and pasta cannot be eaten. Nowadays, there are many gluten free products available in all supermarkets. Careful thought and planning needs to be given to the preparation of food in order to avoid contamination, for example, a separate toaster is a sensible precaution to avoid gluten containing crumbs spreading on to gluten free toast.

Parental choice and influence on children's nutrition

Dietary restrictions that are imposed by parents without a medical reason can be problematic. In an extreme case of parent led dietary restriction in Belgium in 2017, a 9-month-old baby died from starvation because of the exclusion of wheat and dairy products (Bulman 2017). The trend for gluten free diets has extended to children but removing gluten from children's diets when they do not have coeliac disease can have a negative impact; it can mean that children do not receive sufficient nutrition. Gluten free products are energy dense, therefore there is an increased risk of weight gain. There is also an unnecessary impairment of the child's quality of life. If parents have concerns about their children's health because of diet, this needs to be medically investigated to ensure that the child has the correct treatment and dietary nutrition (Wilson et al. 2017).

Parents are increasingly choosing veganism for young children and whilst this choice may be contentious, there is agreement from dietitians that children over two years of age can receive the correct nutritional requirements from dairy and meat free sources (NHS 2021). However, attention should be paid to the amount of fibre that is in the diet. As with all menu planning, it is important that care is paid to ensure that meals include the necessary nutrients; however, children who are vegan may need supplements such as iodine (Jones-Russell 2021).

Eating disorders

Anorexia, bulimia and anorexia nervosa are eating disorders that can affect children and adolescents. Most eating disorders develop in adolescence, with those aged under 20 making up almost half of all people receiving inpatient treatment for an eating disorder in England (BEAT 2022). Eating disorders are thought to be the third most common chronic illness (after asthma and obesity) in adolescent girls (Yeo and Hughes 2011). About 90% of eating disorders develop in women and girls and most are of normal weight or above (only about 15–20% meet criteria for anorexia nervosa) (NICE 2017). Because of the importance of the family in supporting children with eating disorders, NICE (2022) guidance highlights the importance of family therapy.

The role of professionals in promoting healthy eating

All professionals working with children can contribute to promoting healthy eating and drinking. However, the degree of success can be dependent on the child's age. Practitioners in early childhood and education settings are especially well-placed to make a positive contribution. Tatlow-Golden (2019) summarises the role that early years settings can play in supporting babies and young children to develop a healthy relationship with food. Some of the key points from her research are summarised next.

Food caring practices: what helps – and what doesn't

Adults tend to focus on restrictions, pressure to eat, rewards and encouragement when they want children to learn to eat well, small non-food rewards (e.g., stickers) may help with initial neophobia but should be used with caution. The role that adults can play in modelling positive approaches to eating is important, If children see someone try and overtly enjoy an unfamiliar food, they are more likely to try it.

Summary to this section

Solutions to improving children's nutrition are proving difficult to identify. Although it may seem an obvious choice to increase regulation of the food industry and restrict marketing of what are regarded as foods and drink that are of low nutritional value, the reality is that if such foods were not available, it is likely that more children would be hungry. Some families are unable to access fresh food with high nutritional value and may lack the necessary facilities.

Oral health

Poor oral health, leading to dental decay is a mostly preventable physical health condition that can have a profound impact on children's health and wellbeing, both in childhood and across the lifespan. The British Dental Association (BDA) estimates that between 25% and 40% of 5 year olds across the UK have tooth decay, and the impact of lockdown has meant that fewer children will have accessed dental health care and therefore the number will have increased (BDA 2021). For adolescents, it is estimated that 44% have tooth decay, and this number increases to 77% of 15 year olds in Northern Ireland. In England, children from deprived areas living in poverty experience twice the level of dental decay compared to children in less deprived areas (Public Health England 2019). The impact of poor oral health and dental decay can have significant impact on children's day to day lives, causing pain, school absence and loss of sleep. In turn, these can impact on children's behaviour, making them irritable and less able to concentrate. The presence of tooth decay can often be a sign that parents ned support or can be a sign of general neglect (Goodson and Seymour 2019).

Dental decay is completely avoidable for most children, an exception being children with complex medical needs or special educational needs. Children receiving medication for some long-term health conditions such as epilepsy may have side effects which can include gum disease leading to poor oral health. However, for most children, this is not the case. But ensuring that children have good oral health depends on adults (including parents, carers and educators) understanding what needs to be done to keep children's teeth and gums healthy. This contribution highlights how practitioners in early childhood education and care settings.

Promoting good oral health

Keeping children's teeth and gums healthy are reliant on a diet of food and fluids which does not include excessive amounts of sugar. A diet that helps to keep and promote oral health includes crunchy and firm but nutritional foods such as raw carrots and apples. Good oral health relies on introducing the habit of toothbrushing into daily routines at an early age, ideally when the first deciduous ('milk') tooth starts to emerge at about the age of 6 months. In addition to a healthy diet and toothbrushing, visits to dentists are helpful, an examination of a child's teeth by a dentist can help to identify the early stages of dental decay. In England, dental care is a free service to children from the age of two.

Effects of poor oral health

Despite the amount of information about the importance of a healthy diet, regular and effective toothbrushing from babyhood and free dental care, poor dental health is a significant cause of concern. The BDA (2021) highlight the dangers to children's health and state that there needs to be a focus on preventing poor oral health in the same way as there is on addressing obesity in childhood.

If teeth are left to decay, as well as experiencing pain, inadequate nutrition can contribute to other health problems such as weight. There is also an association with speech, language, and communication difficulties. This association can be because of a lack of crunchy, healthy foods in the diet, such as carrots, mastication of such foods helps to develop jaw muscles which are required for speech development. The physical impact of poor oral health can cause emotional difficulties because children can become victims of bullying because of their appearance, which of course has an impact on emotional wellbeing and mental health. Neglecting oral health can lead to decayed, broken, missing and unsightly teeth, which have been found to have a negative impact on a person's ability to find employment (BDA 2018).

Hospital treatment for dental decay

Dental decay is a significant reason that children are admitted to hospital, thus, they are having an anaesthetic and surgery which is completely avoidable. Not only is this unnecessary expense for the NHS, but very importantly this has an impact on children's mental health because admitting a child to hospital and enduring a painful procedure is an example of how a physical condition can have an impact on wellbeing and a child's mental health.

Research focus

Goodwin et al (2015) conducted research in six hospitals in the north west of England involving 456 respondents; the average age of the children in the study was 6.78 years old and the average number of teeth extracted ranged from one to full clearance. The average time from referral to the hospital for the operation to remove the decayed teeth was 137 days, thus children were experiencing discomfort and pain during this period. While removal of decayed teeth is vital, especially if abscesses or infections are present, the long-term considerations of the impact on children of a hospital stay and a general anaesthetic must be considered. In Goodwin et al.'s study, it was noted that 22% of the children referred for tooth extraction had relevant medical history that could have contributed to their dental decay but were not necessarily the main cause of the dental delay. Such medical issues included children who had heart disease, cleft palate, cerebral palsy, behavioural and learning difficulties and allergy to antibiotics. A significant number, 12–37% had been admitted for extractions previously, thus highlighting that dental extraction for decay in some children is a recurring problem.

What can be done to avoid tooth decay?

There is a pressing need to address the causes of poor oral health and to work with children and families to develop sustainable, realistic, and affordable ways of preventing poor oral health. Such interventions include looking at ways of making toothbrushing equipment available and affordable. The BDA highlight the need for marketing strategies that promote the importance of dental checks for young children. Increasing adults' knowledge about healthy eating and drinking and addressing ways to introduce healthy options that contribute to good oral health and hygiene can make a positive contribution. Some families, especially families who may move from home to home regularly, may be described as 'hard to reach'; however, services such as dentists can be hard to reach for some families.

Education settings

Education settings can be a place where health can be promoted, and Early Childhood Education and Care practitioners working in pre-school nursery settings are especially well-placed to promote good oral health. The provision of healthy food and drink, which in England's Early Years Foundation Stage (Department for Education 2021) is a statutory requirement and can make a significant contribution to the healthy development of babies' and children's oral health. Practitioners have the capacity to build good relationships with parents which are critical to identifying, implementing and evaluating effective ways of promoting children's health (Musgrave and Payler 2021) and this can embrace oral health. For professionals working with children, there is a responsibility to address the oral health, especially when teeth become decayed; however, this requires great sensitivity because such conversations with parents, like the treatment of tooth extraction, can be as Goodwin et al. (2015) point out an emotive and contentious issue.

Early childhood settings

The statutory curriculum for children aged 0–5 years in England requires nurseries to take responsibility for children's oral health, it states in the Early Years Foundation Stage (DfE 2021) that 'providers **must** promote the good health, including the oral health, of children attending the setting' (p. 31). Therefore, to comply with this statutory requirement and to contribute to children's good oral health, it is important that they know why and how to do this, and how to work with parents to ensure children have good levels of oral health to avoid short- and long-term damage to physical and mental health.

The following case study explains how Juweirya, a practitioner working in an early years setting, has approached this requirement.

Case study: oral health in early years settings

As children are still coping with the new transition to different rooms, we felt it was very important that we created a warm loving environment where children are taught how to regulate their emotions, understand behavioural expectations and create strong bonds between the practitioners and children before we engage in such an important topic. As we feel this is the basis to then be able to introduce important topics such as oral health.

The introduction of oral health in preschool has begun by bringing awareness to oral health language and vocabulary such as germs, healthy gums, unhealthy gums.

We implement strategies such as reading stories and singing songs about oral health which will help children gain more knowledge of oral health and help to create opportunities to discuss oral health. We hope this will encourage them to take care of their mouths. We will then start to incorporate activities such as brushing teeth, brushing away germs and building a mouth using papier-mache so children become familiar with the different components of the mouth. Also changing our role play into a dentist. This will support children's understanding of oral health.

Comment

In Juweiriya's example, she has drawn upon the broad and deep knowledge of early childhood practice. She has highlighted the need to use appropriate language that is suitable to the age and stage of development of the child. She has also developed an activity that has engaged the children's interest. She has reflected on the success of the activity in relation to teaching the children and reflected on the impact of her own learning and how this contributes to promoting children's oral health. She has demonstrated that she has the confidence to lead the children in the activity as well as negotiating with colleagues to carry out the activity. Replicating this activity in a different context with older age groups may be challenging because of different priorities or a lack of resources; however, this is an example of how a professional has extended her role to consider the holistic health needs of children.

Summary

Poor oral health is a physical condition which can impact on children's physical and mental health. The impact of dental decay can have far reaching effects on physical, cognitive, social and emotional development. The effects can cause school absences and in young children can impact on their school readiness. The school absences can in turn impact on parents, especially those who may need to take time off work or find childcare arrangements while their child is away from education because of their dental problems. The impact of poor oral health and dental decay can have a negative impact on health and employment across the lifespan.

The incidence of dental decay in young children and the long wait time from referral to admission to hospital for children require urgent attention. There is an imperative to find ways to educate adults to understand how to select effective measures to promote good oral health that are embedded in daily routines. Such approaches require the cooperation and willingness of children and parents, and professionals need to be aware of the reasons why some parents may not have been able to incorporate effective toothbrushing, healthy eating and drinking and regular visits to dentists into their routines.

References

BBC News (2021) Pret allergy death: parents welcome Natasha's allergy law. Available from https://www.bbc.co.uk/news/uk-58756597, accessed 6 March 2022.

Beat eating disorders (2022) Information and support. Available from https://www.nice.org.uk/guidance/ng69/chapter/Recommendations#identification-and-assessment, accessed 10 March 2022.

Bennett, V. (2018) Breastfeeding mums can get advice through Alexa. *Nursing Children and Young People* 30(3).

Bentley, J. (2015) The role of vitamin D in infants, children and young people. *Nursing Children and Young People*, 27(1): 28–35.

British Dental Association (2018) Children's oral health in Northern Ireland. Available from https://bda.org/news-centre/blog/Documents/Briefing-Child-oral-health-Northern-Ireland-March-2018.pdf, accessed 10 March 2022.

British Dental Association (2021) Children's oral health: why new obesity programmes are not enough. Available from https://bda.org/news-centre/blog/childrens-oral-health-why-new-obesity-programmes-are-not-enough, accessed 10 March 2022.

Bulman, M. (2017) Baby fed 'alternative' diet weighed less than 10 pounds when he died with totally empty stomach. *The Independent*.

Department for Education (2021) Statutory framework for the Early Years Foundation Stage: setting the standards for learning, development and care for children from birth to five. Available from https://assets.publishing.service.gov.uk/government/uploads/system/uploads/attachment_data/file/974907/EYFS_framework_-_March_2021.pdf, accessed 5 June 2021.

Ek, I. and Hoglund, A. (2016) An experience based treatment for children unwilling to eat. *Nursing Children and Young People* 28(5): 22–28.

Godson, J. and Seymour, D. (2019) Primary preventions and health promotion in oral health. In Emond, A. (Ed) *Health for All Children* (5th Ed). Oxford: Oxford University Press.

Gov.Uk Defra in the news (2021) Natasha's Law comes into force . Available from https://deframedia.blog.gov.uk/2021/10/01/natashas-law-comes-into-force/

Goodwin, M., Sanders, C., Davies, G. et al. (2015) Issues arising following a referral and subsequent wait for extraction under general anaesthetic: impact on children. *BMC Oral Health* 15(3). doi:10.1186/1472-6831-15-3

Gupta, R. S. et al. (2007) Time trends in allergic disorders in the UK. *Thorax* 62(1): 91–96.

HENRY. (2022). Healthy start, brighter future. Available from https://www.henry.org.uk/, accessed 28 May 2020.

Her Majesty's Revenue and Customs (2021) Business tax- Soft drinks industry levy: detailed information. Available from Business tax: Soft Drinks Industry Levy – detailed information – GOV.UK (www.gov.uk), accessed 6 March 2022.

HM Treasury (2018) Soft drinks industry levy comes into effect.

Howell, K. and Musgrave, J. (2021) *A Real Thirst*. Nursery World.

Jones-Russell, M. (2021) *Going Vegan. Nursery World*. London: Mark Allen Publishing.

Marrs, T. and Lack, G. (2013) Why do few food-allergic adolescents treat anaphylaxis with adrenaline? – Reviewing a pressing issue. *Pediatric Allergy and Immunology* 24(3): 222–229.

McMillan, M. (2012) The Nursery School. Original published in 1919 J. M. Dent and Sons: London. Reprinted by Forgotten Books 2012. www.forgottenbooks.com

Meizi, H., Tucker, P. Irwin, J. D., Gilliland, J., Larsen, K., and Hess, P. (2012) Obesogenic neighbourhoods: the impact of neighbourhood restaurants and convenience stores on adolescents' food consumption behaviours. *Public Health Nutrition* 15 (12): 2331–2339.

Musgrave, J. (2014) How do practitioners create inclusive environments for children with chronic health conditions? An exploratory case study. Available from http://etheses.whiterose.ac.uk/6174/1/Jackie%20Musgrave%20-%20Final%20Thesis%20incl%20Access%20Form%20for%20submission%2019-5-14.pdf

Musgrave, J. and Payler, J. (2021) Proposing a model for promoting children's health in early childhood education and care settings. *Children and Society* 35(5): 766–783. https://onlinelibrary.wiley.com/doi/full/10.1111/chso.12449

Narzisi, K. and Simons, J. (2020). Interventions that prevent or reduce obesity in children from birth to five years of age: a systematic review. *Journal of Child Health Care (Early access)*. doi:10.1177/1367493520917863

National Institute for Health and Care Excellence (2014) Vitamin D: supplement use in specific population groups. Available from Overview | Vitamin D: supplement use in specific population groups | Guidance | NICE, accessed 15 January 2022.

National Institute for Health and Care Excellence (2017) Eating disorders: recognition and treatment. published May 2017.

National Institute for Health and Care Excellence (2020) Eating disorders: recognition and treatment. Available from https://www.nice.org.uk/guidance/ng69/chapter/Recommendations# identification-and-assessment, accessed 10 March 2022.

NHS (2020) Planning your pregnancy. Available from Planning your pregnancy - NHS (www. nhs.uk), accessed 6 March 2022.

Newton-Snow, T. (2017) Childhood obesity: can nurses balance the scales? *Nursing Children and Young People* 29(1): 10–11.

Office for Health Improvement and Disparities (2022) Childhood obesity: applying all our health. Updated 7 April 2022.

Public Health England (2015) Child oral health: applying all our health. Available from https:// www.gov.uk/government/publications/child-oral-health-applying-all-our-health/child-oral-health-applying-all-our-health, accessed 27 august 2021.

Public Health England (2019) National Dental Epidemiology Programme for England: oral health survey of 5 year olds 2019.

Public Health England (2017) New survey of mums reveals perceived barriers to breastfeeding.

Royal College of Paediatrics and Child Health (2020) *State of Child Health*. London: RCPCH. Available at: stateofchildhealth.rcpch.ac.uk

Shackleton, N., Milne, B. J., Audas, R., Derraik, J. G. B., Zhu, T., Taylor, R. W., Morton, S. M. B., Glover, M., Cutfield, W. S., and Taylor, B. (2018). Improving rates of overweight, obesity and extreme obesity in New Zealand 4-year-old children in 2010–2016. *Pediatric Obesity*, 13(12): 766–777. 10.1111/ijpo.12260

Tatlow-Golden, M. (2019) 'Big, strong and healthy'? Children, food and eating in the early years, and the role preschools can play. Occasional paper: TACTYC. Available from https:// tactyc.org.uk/wp-content/uploads/2019/01/Occasional-Paper-11-Tatlow-Golden.pdf

Tatlow-Golden and Boyland (2021) Unhealthy digital food marketing to children in the Philippines. Available from unicef-philippines-marketing-report.pdf, accessed 19 March 2022.

Thornton, J. (2019). What's behind reduced child obesity in Leeds? *The British Medical Journal News Analysis*. Published 3 May 2019.

Trower, A. and Gettings, S. (2015) Use of a food allergy care management pathway in adolescents. *Nursing Children and Young People* 27(5): 16–20.

UK Parliament (2021) Event summary: food insecurity and children's health. Available from https://post.parliament.uk/event-summary-food-insecurity-and-childrens-health/#:~:text= According%20to%20the%20UK%20latest,consequences%20for%20children's%20educational%20attainment, accessed 4 February 2022.

Warren, J. (2018) An update on complementary feeding. *Nursing Children and Young People* 30(6): 38–47.

Wilson, E., Gil-Zaragozano, E., and Paul, S. P. (2017) Dangers of a gluten free diet for non-coeliac children. *Nursing Children and Young People* 29(8): 14.

World Health Organisation (2022) Complementary feeding. Available from Complementary feeding (who.int), accessed 16 January 2022.

Yeo, M. and Hughes, E. (2011) Focus Adolescent health: eating disorders – early identification in general practice. Available from http://www.maudsleyparents.org/images/Australian_ family_physician_.pdf, accessed 10 March 2022.

Further resources

Association for Child and Adolescent Mental Health (ACAMH).

NHS (2021) The vegan diet: eat well. Available from https://www.nhs.uk/live-well/eat-well/the-vegan-diet/, accessed 7 March 2022.

10 Caring for children's health and wellbeing

Introduction

This book has explored a range of contemporary issues relating to children's health and wellbeing. For example, in Chapter 8, some of the ways that children can be kept healthy were highlighted, such as preventing some of the causes of ill-health by health promotion activities. Or as discussed in Chapter 5, it was shown how improving children's wellbeing can help children to develop good mental health. This chapter examines the ways that the people in children's lives who have a responsibility to care for their health and wellbeing do so. How adults in the family, as well as in society, deliver care for children's health and wellbeing can be examined through different lenses which include the following:

- The family, which includes parents and children
- Health professionals and practitioners: community and hospital
- The wider community: neighbourhood, schools
- Charities and the voluntary sector – hospices; end-of-life care.

This chapter will explore some of the factors that can influence how parents and professionals fulfil their responsibility to care for children's health and wellbeing. There are a number of contexts where children receive health support and treatment, these will be described, as well as the professionals who provide the health care.

Who gives health care to children?

The individuals who care for children's health and wellbeing include parents and family, or others such as foster parents; health professionals including doctors, nurses, therapists; health care is also provided in education settings including early years pre-school settings, schools and colleges. People working in charitable organisations play a significant role in supporting children's health and wellbeing and can range from global organisations providing health relief in war-torn countries to people working in small, local charities. Figure 10.1 illustrates the different people who can be involved in supporting children's health.

The responsibility can transfer from one person to another as the child moves from one context to another. For example, parents or carers may be responsible overall for children's health, but this can transfer to the education setting for the duration of their attendance. The amount and the type of health support and care a child requires will

DOI: 10.4324/9781003255437-13

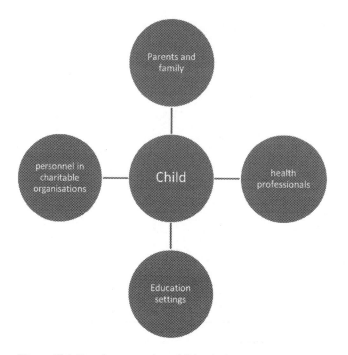

Figure 10.1 People supporting children's health and wellbeing.

partly depend on their individual needs. For example, a child with complex medical needs is likely to require 24-hour health support from parents, with an input from a range of health professionals on a daily basis in the child's education setting as well as input from professionals in health settings. Children with complex medical needs often have their health supported by those working for charitable organisations, such as palliative care in children's hospices.

Age and stage of development

How much parents and other carers work with children to teach them about promoting health and managing their health will partly depend on their age and stage of development. The ideal being that children are taught about health promotion and healthy living from an early age, and as their knowledge increases, they may be able to take greater responsibility for their health. Health is mostly a parental responsibility, unless children are removed from parental care and need the protection of the state, in England, the term used is 'looked-after' children (LAC).

The following section summarises points relating health and how the responsibility can shift as the child becomes older.

Infants and young children's health is partly the role of midwives, health visitors and school nurses. Staff in pre-school and school settings also have a responsibility for children's health. Practitioners in Early Childhood Education and Care settings have a significant role in promoting children's health (Musgrave and Payler 2021). Infants are capable of learning from birth, and children from a very young age can be taught positive messages. Children with chronic and complex medical conditions will require ongoing support with their health, and it is important to be aware that children from a very young age can play an active role in managing their health condition (Musgrave 2014).

Middle childhood

School-aged children's health is part of the responsibility of school nurses and is in a unique position to support children's health and wellbeing. Children in this age group are highly capable of understanding and managing some aspects of their health.

Adolescence in the UK, young people can receive health care in a children's setting up until their 19th birthday. However, it is not always the case that such knowledge and understanding is available as demonstrated by Dr Valentina Baltag, an expert in adolescent health at the World Health Organisation who says, 'it is unacceptable that students of medical and nursing schools leave their training with no understanding of the specific challenges faced by adolescents in accessing healthcare', thus highlighting the need for all health-care providers and support staff to be trained in adolescent health. However, it is not only the responsibility of health care providers to understand adolescent health, education, youth and social care professionals, all who have a responsibility to understand the needs of adolescents and their specific health needs.

Maintaining confidentiality in relation to what an adolescent may tell you about their health requires particular skills. In England, people from the age of 16 can give their medical consent to procedures; however, if a younger person is assessed to be capable of understanding the implications of their decisions, they are deemed to be Gillick competent.

Useful guidance on children and young people's ability to make their own decisions is given in the Fraser guidelines, which were produced following the Gillick case in 1982 (NSPCC 2018). This was a landmark case in which a mother (Victoria Gillick) attempted to stop doctors from giving contraceptive advice to children under the age of 16. In 1985, the High Court dismissed the case, but guidelines were subsequently drawn up by Lord Fraser, where he made an important point about children's rights:

> parental right yields to the child's right to make his own decisions when he reaches a sufficient understanding and intelligence to be capable of making up his own mind on the matter requiring decision.
>
> (NSPCC 2018, p. 2)

A test of 'Gillick competency' means that, if the child understands the advice given, and is mature enough to understand what is involved, then the child has the right to confidentiality. Research by Coyne et al. (2014) suggests that children are not always involved in decisions about their medical care, especially if the illness is serious, when treatment is seen as something that has 'got to be done'. The study pointed out that adolescents were allowed to make some choices but that these did not relate to health decisions such as life-saving treatment.

There may be a fine balance between how, on one hand, one maintains the confidence of an adolescent who may have great insight into the management and consequences of living with a chronic condition and, on the other, how one ensures that an adolescent, who is still legally regarded as being vulnerable, is safeguarded.

Caring for children's health in different contexts

There are different ways that children's health services are organised, and there is not one model that is applicable in a global context. Low-income countries are less likely to have a centrally governed and funded health service for children. How health services are provided can be influenced by many factors, and charities can play an important part in caring for children's health, such as the provision of immunisations to prevent infectious diseases. In Chapter 2, the global influences on health highlighted the combination of factors that can mean providing good health care for children is extremely challenging. In many countries of the world, information relating to providing health care to children relies on being able to access written information. However, it is not unusual for illiteracy levels to be high, and in some communities, there may not be a written language. This means that communication can be a challenge. In many low-income countries, health care that is provided by workers in remote villages who have limited medical equipment and resources can be the norm. In contrast, in many high-income countries, there is a sophisticated system of health care in different settings provided by a range of health specialists available to children.

Providing healthcare in a high-income country

The medical knowledge and advances that have, and continue to be developed, have influenced the treatments that are available to prevent and treat many health conditions. Alongside this, in a high-income country like the UK, this has resulted in a range of different health care settings which have distinct roles in relation to the level of care they provide. Along with the range of settings that provide health care, there has been a range of professionals who specialise in supplying different aspects of healthcare-related roles. In high-income countries, the organisation of children's health is often better funded and likely to have a structure. To use England as an example, children's health services are organised in the following structure. Table 10.1 offers a summary of how health care is organised in the UK.

The following sections explore some of the health care that is provided in each of the different levels of service and settings.

Primary health care

In the UK, children's health care starts when the mother's pregnancy is confirmed; there is free ante-natal care available and the aim of this care to maximise the health of the mother and baby, as well as doing all that can be done to ensure that there is a safe delivery of a baby, or babies, at full term of gestation (40 weeks), who are a healthy weight, with a mother who is also safe and in good health following the delivery. Much of the ante-natal care is coordinated in primary health care settings, such as in a medical centre, where midwives and general practitioners (GPs) monitor pregnancy. Some births that are regarded as being low risk may take place in the mother's home, however many mothers have their baby delivered in a secondary care setting, such as maternity unit in a local hospital. If a pregnancy is not straightforward and especially if a baby is diagnosed with a condition that is predicted to affect their health, tertiary health settings are vital to be able to provide specialist neo-natal care, either in baby units or in paediatric intensive care units (PICUs) that are situated in children's

Table 10.1 Example of healthcare provision for children in a high-income country

Level of health service	Definition	Services available	Professionals
Primary health services	Community based, the first level of health service available to all children health promotion, acute and chronic care	Treatment for minor conditions Ante-natal care Baby clinics Pharmacy	General Practitioner (GP); Speech and Language Therapists (SALT); Health Visitors; Practice Nurses; School Nurses Pharmacists physiotherapists
Secondary Care	Health care that requires more specialised knowledge or equipment	Hospital care including specialist care for chronic health conditions, surgery; diagnostic services such as scans and X-rays	A named paediatrician for each child; surgeons; anaesthetists; medical specialist doctors; physiotherapists Sonographers; radiographers
Tertiary health care	Specialist children's hospitals	Paediatric intensive care units Intensive neonatal care	All of the above plus hospital play therapists; occupational therapists
Palliative health care	*Palliative care for children is the active total care of the child's body, mind and spirit, and also involves giving support to the family. It begins when illness is diagnosed, and continues regardless of whether or not a child receives treatment directed at the disease* (WHO 1998a)	Can be for children with a life-limiting or life-threatening condition, care can be in a hospital, a hospice or the child's home	Specialist nurses; physiotherapists

hospitals. The health care before and immediately after birth is provided by a midwife and if all is well, the care of the newborn is handed over to a Health Visitor after 10 days.

In the UK, children are entitled to be registered with a GP who works in a medical centre. This means that children have the right to healthcare, this healthcare is aimed at preventing health conditions, such preventative health care is coordinated by Registered Health Visitors. Health Visitors work to implement the aims of the Healthy Child Programme; pregnancy and the first 5 years (HCP) (Department of Health 2009a). The aims of the HCP are to prevent some of the causes of poor health and to offer early intervention to infants, children and their parents by providing universal services.

There is also a Healthy Child Programme for children aged 5–19 years (Department of Health 2009b), the aims are again to prevent poor health and provide services for all children that promote good health. The aims of the programme are relevant to the school nurse service (please note that the Healthy Child Programme was updated by Public Health England in March 2021, see reference for the link).

GPs are medically trained doctors who are trained to diagnose and treat a wide range of medical conditions. Therefore, the treatment of acute conditions, such as short-lived viral or bacterial infections are managed by GPs. Chronic health conditions are often managed within general practice. If children require minor surgery or tests to aid diagnosis, GPs are likely to refer children on to secondary care, which can be a local hospital which has a dedicated children's ward.

Practice Nurses work in medical centres alongside GPs and HVs, they can be involved in the provision of health care to children by giving immunisations to babies and children. They have an important role in promoting awareness of the importance of preventing infectious diseases. This role can be fulfilled by coordinating immunisations clinics and educating parents about the need to protect children from potentially life-threatening, but mostly preventable diseases. The approach a practice nurse takes to the administration of immunisations can be critical to how parents take up the offer of immunisations for their children.

School and Public Health Nurses are specially trained to promote the health of children in schools and to work as part of a multi-disciplinary team to deliver the aims of the Healthy Child Programme 5–19. For more about their role, see the School Nurses' Toolkit (Royal College of Nursing 2017).

Secondary and tertiary children's health care

Children's health is best managed where possible by parents in the home and local community with the support of other professionals. However, this ideal is not always feasible or safe. For very young children, hospital care is required, the incidence of hospital admissions is greater for children who live in poverty. Children may need hospital admission because of injuries received either as an accident, or non-accidental, injury, or to receive treatment for a medical emergency. Depending on the nature of the reason, a child may be referred to secondary medical care at a local hospital. In England, part of the National Service Framework guidance (Department of Health 2004) states that children should be treated in separate units away from adults.

Historical perspective: the care of children in hospitals

In England, hospitals which were dedicated to the care of children were opened about 150 years ago because the urbanisation of city areas and the heavy industry that had developed meant that children's health was negatively impacted upon by poor air quality and the high risk of infectious diseases. In Birmingham, the Children's Hospital was opened in one of the poorest areas, consequently, there are still hospitals in most of the big, formerly industrial manufacturing cities. At the time that children's hospitals were opened, the medical care that was available was basic, it was going to be many years until safe general anaesthesia and surgical techniques were to be developed; the medications that are routinely available to manage chronic health conditions, such as insulin for diabetes, were similarly years away from being discovered. Consequently, until the middle of the last century, if children became unwell, there was little that could be done to cure them. The main benefit to children of being in hospital was that they could receive nursing care and rest in a clean environment where they were supplied with nutritious food. It was more often the expectation that children would not survive. Children who did survive dangerous illnesses, usually spent long periods of time in hospital convalescing. The expectation that children may not survive, and the difficulties associated with visiting children in hospital, shaped the way that the care of children in hospital developed. It became the norm that children would be admitted to hospital and left in the care of nurses, sometimes for many months, and parents were dissuaded from visiting their children. This situation persisted until the middle of the last century and only changed as a consequence of the work of the Robertsons and the review of the care of children in hospital (Platt Report 1959).

The influence of the Robertson on the care of children in hospital

The post-second world war period was a time of increased awareness of the potential impact of attachment theory and the links with children's wellbeing and mental health. Joyce and James Robertson researched the effects of separation form her mother on a 2 years old called Laura. Their observations of Laura's behaviour were filmed. It was perhaps surprising that Laura responded by becoming withdrawn and appeared compliant, rather than being overtly distressed. The findings from the Robertson's research contributed to a change in national policy to the way that children were cared for in hospital.

At the time I started my nurse training, some of the sisters in charge of the ward were still approaching the care of children in hospital in the same ways as before the Robertson's work was published. The following words are from my Masters dissertation, which focussed on the emotional needs of babies (Musgrave 2009), this extract is where I drew on my nursing experience and reflected on my motivation to research this subject.

Personal reflection

A powerful example of what was to become my motivation to work with children, and eventually formed the basis of my interest in babies. There was a 12-month-old baby, I can't remember his name. He had been on the ward for several days and had not received visitors. He had a brain tumour which had been operated on, but the operation had not been successful, and he was terminally ill. He had a big bandage on his head, and he was mostly unresponsive and lay in the cot and was twitching from time to time. I was allocated to care for him on the day that would turn out to be his last day of living. I was concerned about his twitching, so I got him out of his cot and I swaddled him in one of the hospital blankets and gently hugged him close. I thought that this seemed to soothe him, the twitching stopped, but it may well have been more about making me feel better. I felt desperate that this baby was dying in a bleak hospital room without parents or a family member being present. After about 20 minutes, the staff nurse came in to the side room and she told me to put the baby back in his cot and go to help the other staff to serve the children their evening meal. When I pointed out that the baby seemed calmer when he was being held, she responded that I 'couldn't just sit down all day' and it was my duty to help colleagues.

When I returned to him, after completing the menial task I had been sent to do, he had died, alone.

Comment

The feelings that this incident provoked in me were so strong, I felt as if I had let this baby down. I couldn't tell if he was in pain and of course, I had no idea whether he was in any way aware of what was going on, although I guess that as he was soothed by being held, he must have had some feelings. As the years have gone by, I found myself becoming more disturbed by the incident and I felt a need to try and find out an explanation for the nursing care that was given to a terminally ill child who did not have family around him.

At the time that I was a junior student nurse in 1979, some of the sisters who managed the wards had trained many years previously and had adopted the practices of their time which pre-dated the pioneering work of the Robertsons, which is described more below.

Menzies-Lyth's (1960) study explored some of the possible reasons that nurses demonstrated a lack of emotional involvement in the care of patients. She identified that one cause was that nurses were trying to avoid the pain and distress, caused by the breaking of relationships with patients. In the experience that I cite, the death of a baby would cause the breaking of the relationship. With the passage of time, I can understand that practice reflected the beliefs of that time, which was that it was important 'not to get emotionally involved' with patients, partly because it protected the nurses from emotional pain as a consequence of the death of a patient. This belief was reinforced by senior to junior nursing staff until research, such as Menzies-Lyth's and the Robertsons, helped to change understanding and practice. I can also understand why leaving the baby to die on his own was thought to be the correct approach because little was known at that time about end-of-life care for children; however, the emergence of hospices for children has made end-of-life care more humane.

The children's hospice movement

The first children's hospice was opened in England in 1982 to provide palliative care to children. According to Brown (2007), the philosophy of paediatric palliative care is to 'attend to the psychological, physical, spiritual and social needs of the child and their family' (p. 18) in order to enhance the quality of remaining life.

Working with parents

Parents influence children's health from conception and throughout life. The importance of ante-natal care is discussed in Chapter 3. Some of the health outcomes for children are determined at birth, an infant who is born at full term gestation following a normal delivery into a family who is not living in poverty is more likely to be healthier than infants who are born prematurely, or are light for dates, into a family living in poverty. The country that a child is born into also influences the health outcomes, low income countries are less likely to have health services available, such as organised ante-natal care. In countries with health services available to all, often free such as in the UK, the health outcomes are better. However, there are many other factors that can affect children's health and in turn, this can impact on the way the child is cared for, which in turn influences the health outcomes for children.

Communication with parents

Health can be a sensitive subject for anyone and for parents, their children's health can be especially sensitive. The way that parents are communicated with can influence how receptive parents are to any discussions about their children's health. Any encounter about children's health between parents and professionals who work with children requires tact and diplomacy. This point can be applied to all situations. For example, a teacher may be concerned about a child in their class who has an infestation of headlice, or it can apply to staff on a PICU who are caring for children with complex health needs. In relation to any health situation, parents are likely to feel a range of emotions, such as anxiety and concern. Some parents may become defensive and possibly become angry and aggressive. Evans (2019) highlights that reports relating to controversial complex cases where health staff and parents were in legal dispute about the decisions relating to their child cite poor communication as a contributory factor. Poor communication 'such as conflicting messages being given to families by different members of staff and the use of insensitive language as a major cause of problems' (p. 9).

Parents' role in caring for children's health

Many parents, especially caring for children with chronic and complex health needs can become experts in their child's care because they understand their child and the unique ways that they may respond to ill health. Parents can become advocates for their child's health and will pursue what they feel is the best treatment for their child (Lee and Lynn 2017; Musgrave 2014).

Influences on how families care for their children's health

Throughout this book, there have been examples of factors that can influence how, when and even whether children receive the sort of health care that is available and regarded as the best there can be. A significant influence on how children's health needs are recognised and met depends on the parents' role. Parents can positively or negatively impact on how they support children's health.

Other factors that influence how parents support their children's health include the parents' level of education, some parents may have special educational needs and potentially have limited understanding of the complexities of children's health. Parents may not be literate; therefore, they may have difficulty reading health-related information. Parents may speak the language of the country they are living in. The socio-economic status of the parents can influence the kinds of resources they have access to, living in poverty is regarded as being a negative influence on children's health. If parents are involved in work outside the home, there may be more money available to the family, which can benefit children's health, but on the other hand, there may be less time available to spend in activities that promote children's health.

The family structure and size can also impact on children's health, a child with a chronic health condition can require a great deal of parental time and this in turn can impact on siblings within the family. A child who is 'looked-after' by the state and not living with their biological parents may have moved between homes and there may not be a record of health-related activities. Keeping track of a child's immunisation record can be a challenge at the best of times, let alone when a child has lived with several different adults at several addresses.

The cultural beliefs or practices of the community one lives in can impact on health. Culture can be defined as the ideas, customs and beliefs of a particular group of people. Religion is also a powerful influence on beliefs and customs. It is important that as professionals there is a sensitivity and awareness of religious and cultural beliefs. However, it is also vitally important to be absolutely clear about what is legal and illegal in relation to children's health.

Family structure

Traditional definitions of what we mean by the term 'family' need to be put to one side. In many cultures, a family may be defined as being comprised of two parents and children, or a child, living together. However, in modern society, family can be structured very differently, there may be two parents of the same sex, a single parent, a re-constituted family (where parents live together with children from other relationships), or the family may be extended to include other members such as grandparents. Some children are parented by kinship carers, meaning they are blood-related but not the biological parent. And of course, some children are adopted or fostered and parented by adults who have been appointed by the state. The family structure may be a powerful influence on children's health.

Parenting style

As discussed in Chapter 2, the style that adults adopt to parent children in hugely influential on health outcomes. Baumrind in the 1960s described parenting styles that are still referred to. An authoritarian parental style is one where there are strict boundaries and children have limited freedom. This approach can cause rebellion, especially in adolescence and in relation to health it can be a contributory factor to non-compliance with medication.

An authoritative parenting style is one where parents are supportive and nurturing, children are given some agency, but they are aware of boundaries. In relation to children who have an ongoing health condition, this approach can be especially helpful because it allows the child to develop some responsibility in relation to managing their health. Parents who have a permissive approach may be less inclined to expect their children to take responsibility, there may be loose boundaries. Parents may find it difficult to say no and this may result in a range of health-related issues. For example, boundaries about eating and the amount of screen time may not be in place which in turn, may result in unhealthy eating and physical inactivity. Consequently, the parenting style can impact on children's health.

Health condition of children

From the perspective of the child, the kind of health condition that a child may have can also influence how the parents can provide health care. The length of time that a child needs care for and what they need doing to support their health depends to some extent on the condition. A child who has ongoing complex medical needs may require 24-hour care, many of the needs will be provided by the parents in the child's home. A child who has a viral illness will also need support and care from their parents; however, such support is short-lived. A child who has a chronic health condition will require ongoing support from their parents. The following section illustrates some of the ways that a child's chronic health condition may impact on a family. The summary is drawn from my doctoral research.

Research focus: the impact on families of a living with a child with chronic health condition(s)

As discussed in Chapter 8, some of the most common chronic health conditions that affect children include asthma, eczema, diabetes, epilepsy and sickle cell anaemia. The effects of living with a child with a chronic, or more than one, chronic condition can impact upon the child, or young person's family routines in a variety of ways. Depending on the interventions that are required to manage the condition, the impact may be made apparent several times a day. In addition to interventions that are required, there may be restrictions to what the child and the family can do, which can impact upon other siblings. The impact of living in a family with a child who has ongoing chronic health care needs can be financial, social and emotional, and may even be regarded as limiting freedom.

The financial costs that can be associated with having a child with a chronic health condition can arise as a result of the impact on parents' ability to work. A child who needs to attend appointments with medical professionals to receive, or to review, treatment will frequently be taken to such appointments by their parents or other family members. This means that child care for other siblings may have to be organised. For parents who are employed outside the home, absence from work may need to be negotiated and sometimes, parents may miss out on their earnings. In some cases, the care needs may be such that parents find it difficult to balance the demands of employment and the demands of caring for their children's health. If this is the case, financial hardship can be the result. There can cost associated with the management of a child's chronic condition that is not visible. For example, children may need particular foods, clothing or even laundry products to manage the condition, such requirements can be a drain on a family's financial resources.

Parents who participated in my research reported conflicts that had arisen because of the impact of their child's chronic health condition on siblings and the family. They reported that there were emotional effects on siblings because they may feel that the child with the chronic condition takes up more parental time. This can lead to resentment and can be a justifiable feeling because a child who needs medication or health care routines inevitably takes up more parental time and attention. Parents described how the child's chronic condition meant that the family lost the ability to do things in a more spontaneous way. This was because there was a need to make careful plans to ensure that the child's additional health needs were going to be met. Parents described some of the difficulties associated with accessing food when outside the home, this was particularly so in relation to children with potentially life-threatening reactions to food.

Having a child who does not sleep well because of the symptoms of their chronic condition often means that others within the family do not sleep either and inadequate sleep can create difficulties for all members of the family. Parents in my research described how their son only slept for 3–4 hours at a time, he would wake up scratching because of his eczema and one of his parents would need to re-apply cream during the night to soothe his skin. In order to minimise the impact of their son's sleep disturbance on the rest of the family, they would sleep in shifts.

My research highlighted that living with a child with a chronic condition can exert pressure on families, such pressures can be even more profound if there are other factors such as living in poverty. However, what also emerged from the parents in my research was that their children with chronic health conditions can be a source of pride to their families because of the way they respond to and manage their condition.

Parents' involvement in hospital care

Since the publication of the Platt Report (1959) and the subsequent change in practice in hospitals regarding the involvement of parents, there has been a move away from parents being completed excluded from the care of their children towards parents being completely involved in their child's health care. For a short stay in hospital for a routine procedure, this may not be problematic, but for children with long-term and complex conditions, this can be a very intense experience which can have long-term effects. This is especially the case if a child requires care on a PICU.

Caring for children on PICUs

Medical advances have resulted in infants surviving when previously, the presence of some conditions would have meant that either the pregnancy would have miscarried, or the infant would only survive for a short time. Similarly, medical advances have meant that responses to children experiencing physical trauma have a higher chance of survival. PICU is staffed by highly skilled specialists; a child on PICU will be looked after by medical consultants, doctors, specialist nurses, hospital ply therapists, physiotherapists, pharmacists and radiographers. Parents are often entering an alien environment where there is little distinction between night and day, parents are likely to be exhausted. They are observers as their child is cared for by a range of different professionals. The parents will have had to learn a whole new language associated with their child's health situation, possibly struggling with understanding the meaning of what they are being told and grappling with the implications of the information they are being told.

To illustrate some of the complexities, read the case study about Lottie and her family.

Case study: Lottie

Lottie is 2 years old and she is being cared for on the PICU of a Children's Hospital which is 30 miles from where she and her family live. Lottie has two siblings, twin brothers who are 4 years old. Lottie's mum is a childminder and her dad is a self-employed plumber. Lottie was playing in the garden with her brothers and in the few seconds that Lottie's mum had popped into the kitchen to turn the oven off, one of them carried her to the trampoline so that he could jump with her; however, Lottie bounced high and she fell off the trampoline and sustained a brain injury.

Lottie had emergency surgery to remove a blood clot, but the scans and brain tests following the surgery revealed that Lottie is brain injured. She has been on PICU for 10 days and is being ventilated to support her breathing and maintain her airway. Attempts to take her off the ventilator have been unsuccessful. Because the area of her brain which is responsible for breathing has been damaged following the fall. The consultant in charge of Lottie's care is pessimistic about whether she will be able to breathe independently again, meaning that she would need to remain on a ventilator for the rest of her life. The brain damage she has sustained means that she will not respond to any stimulation. If she were to return home, she would require 24-hour care with ventilation and other medical equipment. The PICU team has broached the subject of withdrawing treatment which will mean that Lottie will die.

Questions

*   Having read Lottie's case, can you imagine the emotions that Lottie's parents are experiencing?
*   What are the practical difficulties that they are likely to be experiencing?

Even if you have never had personal experience of being with your child on a PICU, it is hopefully not difficult to imagine some of the parents' emotions during this time. It is likely that they feel as if they are living in a nightmare, they may be in shock, or denial about the situation, they are likely to feel angry about being in the situation. Lottie's mum is likely to be angry and guilty because of the consequences of leaving the children for a tiny amount of time, angry with Lottie's brother for his actions, Lottie's dad is possibly angry with her mum because she left them alone. Many of these emotions are similar to those experienced in response to grief and bereavement. The family is separated, and this is likely to cause anxiety for Lottie's brothers.

From a practical point of view, both parents have been at Lottie's side for most of the time she has been on PICU, returning home to get clothes and to see the boys. Lottie's parents are at the family home to care for the boys and they are trying to keep their routines as normal as possible. Both parents are self-employed and do not earn money if they are not at work and the cost of travelling backwards and forwards, car parking costs and loss of earnings are all becoming an additional concern. It is understandable that such situations can become very tense; as happened in England when there have been highly publicised cases where the decisions of parents of children with complex medical conditions differed to the health professionals who were caring for them.

Complex situations and difficult decisions

There have been some complex situations where disputes have arisen between health professionals and the parents of children who have been cared for on a PICU. Some of these disputes have become legal cases and the number of cases that are reported to the High Court in England is estimated to be about 10. In 2017 and 2018, there were two high-profile cases reported in the media about children who were being kept alive mechanically and receiving treatment on PICUs.

The combination of complex medical cases, difficult and final decisions about care and the negative impact of social media all contributed to inflamed and toxic situations.

Charmian Evans (2017) wrote an article in response to the Charlie Gard's case where she described the death of her 5-year-old son, Guy. He had cerebral palsy after having been resuscitated following what was described as a 'near miss cot death' when he was 4 months old. Evans describes how she hoped that there would be a cure for Guy, to return him to his former level of ability and investigated options of maximising the possibility of this happening, even to the point of considering a move to live in Hungary so Guy could attend the Peto Institute which has a reputation for successful treatment for children with cerebral palsy. However, Guy became unwell with a serious chest infection and even though there may have been treatment that could have kept him alive, such treatment may not have been in Guy's best interests. Despite, the love they had for their son and the knowledge that their lives would never be the same again, Evans and her husband knew that 'sometimes you just have to let them go' (Evans 2017, p. 25).

Impact on parents of caring for a child with very complex medical needs

These contrasting approaches from parents in similar situations illustrate two different responses. Of course, there is no right or wrong way for parents to respond in such circumstances because each case will be unique and so are the individuals involved. Taking a child who needs 24-hour care is a difficult way forward. Lee and Lynn (2017) report on the long-term effects on mental health and wellbeing of parents of children requiring long-term ventilation at home. The findings highlight the ongoing nature of the care that is required, children with complex medical needs may have a range of tubes that require management, for example, feeding tubes, urinary catheters as well as the machinery required to support their child's breathing. Parents are required to learn many clinical skills which need to be carried out around the clock. They report that there is a lack of support that is available for parents; there is limited respite care available to give parents a break. Financial adversity is another concern because it is often the case that at least one parent did not work in paid employment because of the child's medical needs.

Parents reported feelings of social isolation, this was partly because 'it took too much energy to organize simple activities' (ibid, p. 35) consequently, parents tended to remain at home because it required less energy to do so than going out. A lack of sleep, the emotional impact of being responsible for a completely dependent child, financial worries and social isolation all contributed to the parents experiencing poor mental health. On the other hand, for some parents, the task of caring for their child brought them a sense of joy.

For parents who take the option of discontinuing care for their child, they too will experience similar feelings, such as an awareness that their lives will never be the same again. Such decisions are incredibly difficult for all concerned; consequently, the Nuffield Council on Bioethics (2019) has issued guidance to help health professionals who are caring for children who are in similar situations.

Caring for children's health in education settings

All who work with children in education settings have a responsibility to promote children's good health. Health promotion is discussed in more detail in Chapter 4, and the ways that people in education settings can promote health by preventing infection are discussed in detail in Chapter 6. The ways that educators can support children who have a chronic, that is, an ongoing health condition is discussed in Chapter 8. Therefore, the content relating to how educators can care for children's health is focused on some general points, specifically their leadership role in caring for aspects of children's health.

Leadership and children's health

The staff in education settings, practitioners in pre-school settings, and teachers and teaching assistants in schools, are well placed to lead on caring for children's health. They also have a significant responsibility to care for children's health. Supporting a child in emergency situations, administering first aid, or initiating medical help, can cause anxiety because of the responsibility of doing so. In addition, they will be observing the distress of the child, and are likely to be fearful about the outcome. At such a time, it is important that adults remain calm, appear confident and reassuring to all involved, especially to the child.

Educators have a responsibility for the ongoing health of children, for example, ensuring that the food children are offered is healthy, and that the ethos of the setting supports the development of good mental health and wellbeing. Many more children with complex medical conditions are attending mainstream education and children with chronic conditions, such as asthma, require ongoing support. The intersection of children's health and education is a space where roles and responsibilities can overlap, or on the other hand, they may be seen to belong to another professional and therefore, who holds responsibility for certain aspects of caring for children's health can become blurred. Therefore, caring for children's health in education settings can be contentious. It is of course understandable that teachers may feel that some aspects of care are not their responsibility. The reasons why there may be reluctance need to be explored in order to ensure that children receive the heath care they require in order to be able to engage with their education. Reasons for reluctance to engage with some aspects of health care may be because of lack of training, fear of doing something wrong which may damage the child, or even expose the person to legal action. Another reason why educators may find caring for children's health difficult is because of the time they need to devote to teaching children and ensuring they are meeting the aims of the curriculum. Health visitors and school nurses are key health professionals in delivering the aims of the Healthy Child Programme (Department of Health 2009a), but there is a shortage of people in these roles, which has led to insufficient levels of service. This in turn will leave a gap in how children's health care is delivered in pre-school and school settings.

It is vital that children's health is supported in education settings, and such support can be offered by ensuring that policies are developed which help all staff to understand the specific requirements for individual children's health needs as well as all children's health needs.

Education health and care plans

In addition to policies which help to educate staff about the health needs of all and individual children, Education, Health and Care plans help to ensure that all staff have knowledge and understanding of the health needs of children with additional needs. It is a legal requirement in England as part of the Children and Families Act (2014) for an EHC plan to be in place. One of the purposes of the EHC Plan is for it to be a written central point of information for all professionals so that everyone knows the specific actions that are required to be taken to care for the child's health. In some cases where children have died of anaphylaxis, it has been highlighted that a lack of a policy and plan was a contributory factor.

Summary

This chapter has given an overview of how health services and care are delivered to children in a range of contexts. The content highlights the ways that professionals can work together with parents to support and promote children's health.

References

Brown, E., and Warr, B. (2007) *Supporting the Child and Family in Paediatric Palliative Care*. London: Jessica King Publishers.

Children and Families Act (2014) Available from http://www.legislation.gov.uk/ukpga/2014/6/contents/enacted, accessed 19 August 2019.

Coyne, I., Amory, A., Kiernan, G., and Gibson, F. (2014). Children's participation in shared decision-making: Children, adolescents, parents and healthcare professionals' perspectives and experiences. *European Journal of Oncology Nursing*, 18, 273–280. 10.1016/j.ejon.2014.01.006.

Department of Health (2002).

Department of Health (2004) National Service Framework for Children, Young People and Maternity Services.Available from https://assets.publishing.service.gov.uk/government/uploads/system/uploads/attachment_data/file/199952/National_Service_Framework_for_Children_Young_People_and_Maternity_Services_-_Core_Standards.pdf, accessed 24 July 2022.

Department of Health (2009a) The healthy child programme: pregnancy and the first 5 years of life. Available from https://assets.publishing.service.gov.uk/government/uploads/system/uploads/attachment_data/file/167998/Health_Child_Programme.pdf, accessed 19 August 2019.

Department of Health (2009b) Healthy child programme: 5-19. Available from https://assets.publishing.service.gov.uk/government/uploads/system/uploads/attachment_data/file/492086/HCP_5_to_19.pdf, accessed 19 August 2019.

Evans, C. (2017) Sometimes you just have to let them go. *The Sunday Telegraph*. 11 June 2017.

Evans, N. (2019) Advice on resolving disagreements with the families of critically ill children. *Nursing Children and Young People* 31(4): 8–9.

Lee, J. and Lynn, F. (2017) Mental health and wellbeing of parents caring for a ventilator dependent child. *Nursing Children and Young People* 29(5): 33–40.

Menzies-Lyth (1960).

Musgrave, J. (2009) What do students know about babies' emotional needs and development? Unpublished Masters dissertation, University of Sheffield.

Musgrave, J. (2014) How do practitioners create inclusive environments for children with chronic health conditions? An exploratory case study. Thesis for Doctor of Education, University of Sheffield. Available from http://etheses.whiterose.ac.uk/6174/1/Jackie%20Musgrave%20-%20Final%20Thesis%20incl%20Access%20Form%20for%20submission%2019-5-14.pdf

Musgrave, J., and Payler, J. (2021) Proposing a model for promoting Children's Health in Early Childhood Education and Care Settings. *Children & Society*, 35, 766–783. 10.1111/chso.12449.

NSPCC (2018).

Nuffield Council on Bioethics (2019) Briefing note: disagreements on the care of critically ill children. Available from http://nuffieldbioethics.org/wp-content/uploads/Disagreements-in-the-care-of-critically-ill-children.pdf, accessed 6 May 2019.

Platt, H. (1959) *The Welfare of Children in Hospital*. London: Ministry of Health Services Council.

Public Health England (2021) Healthy Child Programme 0–19: health visitor and school nurse commissioning. Available from https://www.gov.uk/government/publications/healthy-child-programme-0-to-19-health-visitor-and-school-nurse-commissioning, accessed 20 August 2022.

Royal College of Nursing (2017) A toolkit for school nurses. Available from file:///C:/Users/jm39645/AppData/Local/Temp/PUB-006316.pdf, accessed 19 August 2019.

World Health Organisation (1998a) Definition of palliative care. Available from https://www.who.int/cancer/palliative/definition/en/, accessed 22 July 2019.

Other resources

Council for Disabled Children (2017) Resources including examples of good practice. Available from https://councilfordisabledchildren.org.uk/search/content/education%20health%20care%20plans, accessed 15 August 2019.

Robertson Films (1952) A 2 year old goes to hospital. Available from https://www.google.co.uk/search?source=hp&ei=oyQ4XaviDMSYlwTwnLaQAw&q=the+robertson+a+2+year+old+goes+to+hospital&oq=the+robertsons+a+2+yea&gs_l=psy-ab.1.0.33i22i29i30l2.1986.9907..12796... 0.0..1.336.2315.17j3j1j1…...0 … .1..gws-wiz … ..0..0i131j0j0i10j0i22i30j0i22i10i30.JCWxQHQ5_wI

11 Summary and concluding thoughts

This book has explored the role that all adults have in supporting and promoting the health of babies, children and young people. The world that we live in is a complex one, and the complexities directly impact on children's physical and mental health.

It is our responsibility as adults to reflect on the way we treat our children, to consider how we can make their world less complex. All children are vulnerable, and we have a duty to protect them. We also have a duty and responsibility to educate them about how they can develop healthy habits right from the start of life. In the period of recovery following the pandemic, some children's mental and physical health will require even more attention and consideration (Figure 11.1).

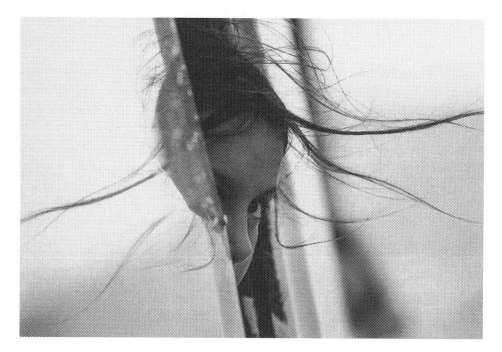

Figure 11.1 Girl looking out of a window.

Credit line: Benjamin Voros – Unsplash Copyright notice: © Benjamin Voros/Unsplash IMG001590.

DOI: 10.4324/9781003255437-14

Having read the book, I urge you to consider the following questions:

1   What are the main learning points you are going to take away from reading this book?
2   Has the content of the book impacted on your thinking?
3   How will you change your practice as a result of engaging with this book?

Many thanks for reading this book, please get in touch with any comments that you may have.

Index

Printed in the United States
by Baker & Taylor Publisher Services